CHAMPNEYS

Spa secrets for body and soul

CHAMPNEYS

Spa secrets for body and soul

Your inspirational seasonal guide including recipes, beauty treatments, fitness tips and well-being trends from the luxury spa experts

By Champneys with Elisabeth Wilson

Copyright © Champneys Henlow Limited, 2009

The right of Champneys Henlow Limited to be identified as the author of this book has been asserted in accordance with the Copyright, Designs and Patents Act 1988.

First published in 2009 by
The Infinite Ideas Company Limited
36 St Giles
Oxford, OX1 3LD
United Kingdom
infiniteideas   www.infideas.com

A CIP catalogue record for this book is available from the British Library

ISBN 978–1–905940–95–0

Brand and product names are trademarks or registered trademarks of their respective owners.

Cover and text designed by Cylinder
Typeset by Cylinder
Exercise illustrations on pages 117–119, 124–125, 193–194 and 252–255 by David Peduzzi
Printed in Italy

Acknowledgements

Every single staff member (past and present) contributes to make Champneys what it is today: one of the most successful, prestigious and popular spa resorts in the UK. For this reason this book would not have been possible without them. However a few special thank yous go to the following individuals who have played an extra special part in making this book come to fruition:

Hilary Dart, Brand Director

Louise Day, Fitness Director

Gary Foster, Head Chef, Champneys Forest Mere

Ailsa Higgins, Champneys Nutritionist

David Melleney, Graphic Design Manager

Jo Parker, Spa Director

Dawn Saunt, PA to Spa Director

Sharon Scott, Marketing Manager

Richard Smith, Head Chef, Champneys Springs

Other special thanks goes to Elisabeth Wilson, Kate Santon, David Peduzzi and Natalie Smith.

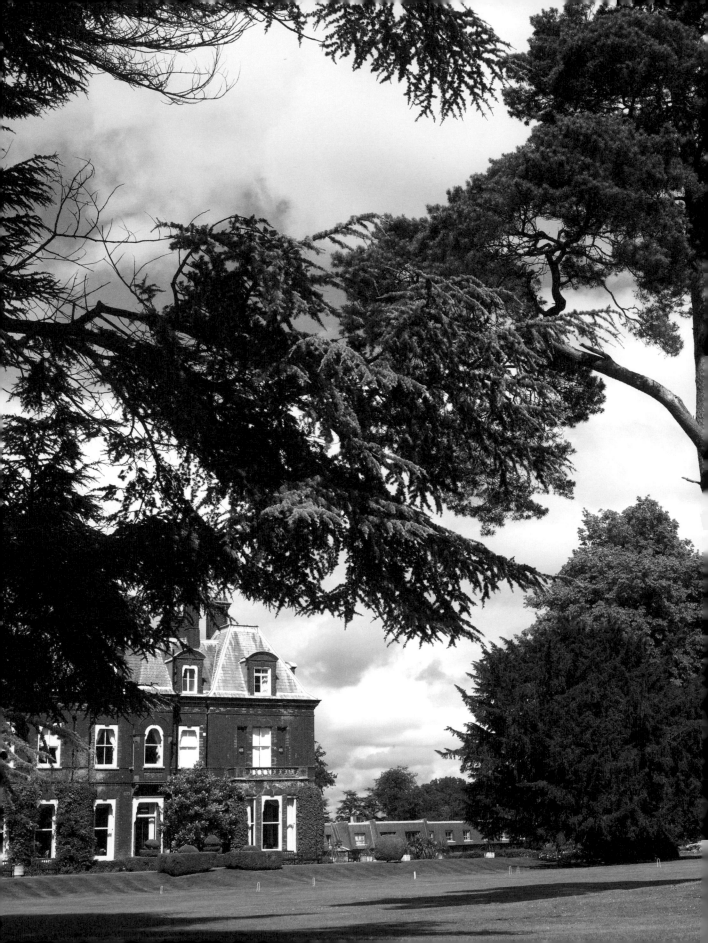

Contents

Foreword vi

Introduction 1

Spring 13

Summer 77

Autumn 153

Winter 221

Index 289

Recipe index 299

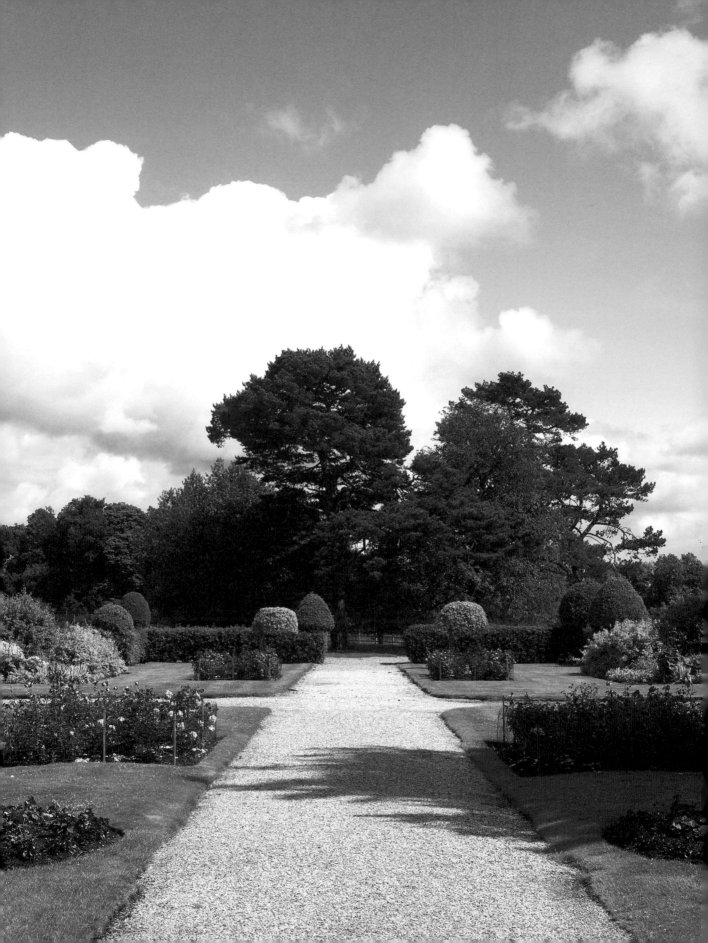

Foreword

Every day, hundreds of guests pass through each one of the four Champneys resorts. We want every one of them to leave feeling fitter, healthier and more deeply inspired to look after their physical and emotional well-being in the future.

This book aims to give you that same Champneys' experience at home.

Our guests choose to visit Champneys to enjoy the peace and calm, to jump-start a fitness programme, to lose a little weight or for relaxation and pampering. We achieve this with luxurious beauty treatments, delicious nutritious meals, superb fitness facilities and holistic well-being services. In this, our season-by-season guide, we have distilled some of that expertise so you can benefit from it at home.

This book is intended to be your companion throughout the year with suggestions tailored to each season. Why? Because our lives follow a natural rhythm. If we want to start getting fit, we will find that we have a special energy and enthusiasm for it in spring, reflecting nature bursting into bloom all around us. In summer, we find it easier to succeed in losing weight when we are naturally drawn to lighter foods and want to get outside to socialise and relax rather than 'hibernating' at home. Autumn, that lovely lull between lazy summer and quiet winter, is the natural time to make the most of the last warm days, get cracking on new projects and turn our attention to how best to conserve our resources and prepare for the coming winter. And it's in winter that we want to retreat into ourselves, take time to dream by the fire, restore ourselves with warm baths scented with fragrant oils, and draw closer to the people that we depend on the most. These rhythms ruled our ancestors' lives for millennia – it's only recently that technology has made them less relevant.

In our Champneys resorts, surrounded by acres of beautiful English countryside, it's easy for guests to remember nature's natural rhythms, which is one of the reasons so many clients find visiting us such a relaxing experience. But, all too often in our busy twenty-first century lives, it's easy to forget the connection to nature. This book aims to give you the breathing space that a trip to Champneys would achieve – and to remind you that by working with each season you can get back in tune with your own internal rhythms, reduce stress, nurture yourself, age-proof your looks and body, and feel and look your best. Whatever your goals for your health and well-being, achieving them becomes a lot easier when you are in tune with both the world outside and your own internal rhythms.

At Champneys, holistic isn't just a word but a way of life. We help our guests to address every aspect of looking and feeling good, and we do the same in our year book. Each season is divided into sections reflecting what we offer guests at our resorts:

- **Eat** – Champneys' approach to healthy nutrition: balance, moderation, variety. This includes 'Inspiration to eat well' – seasonal recipes from the Champneys' chefs.

- **Move** – the information you need from our trainers to restore energy levels and achieve a fit, supple body that will defy ageing.

- **Love yourself** – our famous therapeutic spa beauty treatments adapted for your home.

- **Well-being** – advice from our life coaches and well-being experts on getting the most from your life.

- **Escape** – the distilled essence of our treatment programmes so that you can take time out of your schedule just for you, and effortlessly achieve your health and well-being goals.

We believe that nothing can quite reproduce a visit to one of our resorts. But until we meet you for the first time, or welcome you back for a return visit, we believe our year book will provide you with the next best thing. It is your guide to a happier, healthier, more beautiful way of living.

Stephen Purdew

Director and co-owner of the Champneys group

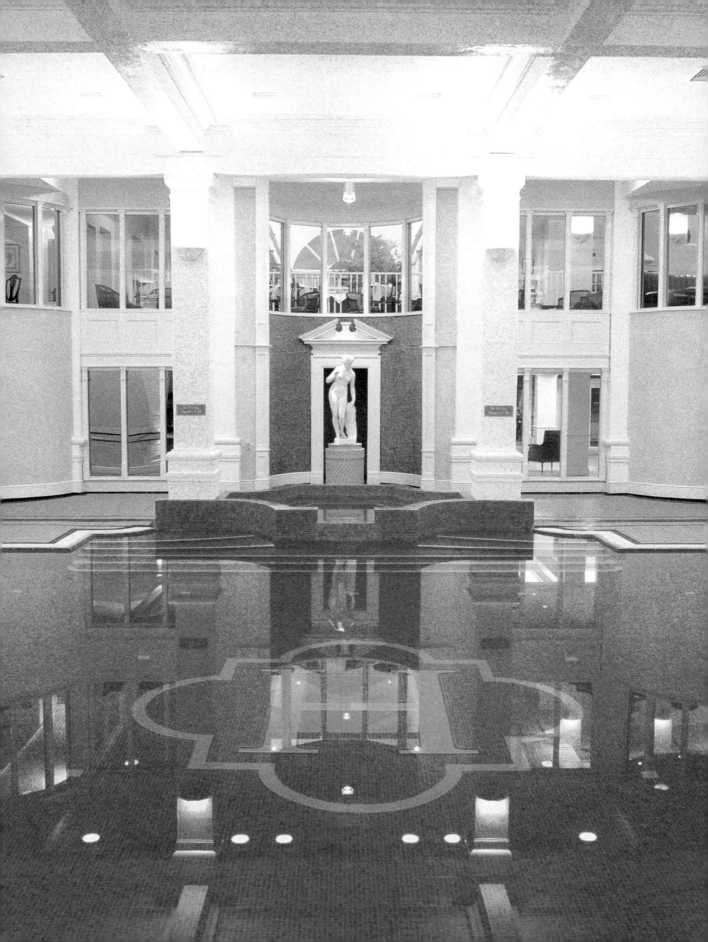

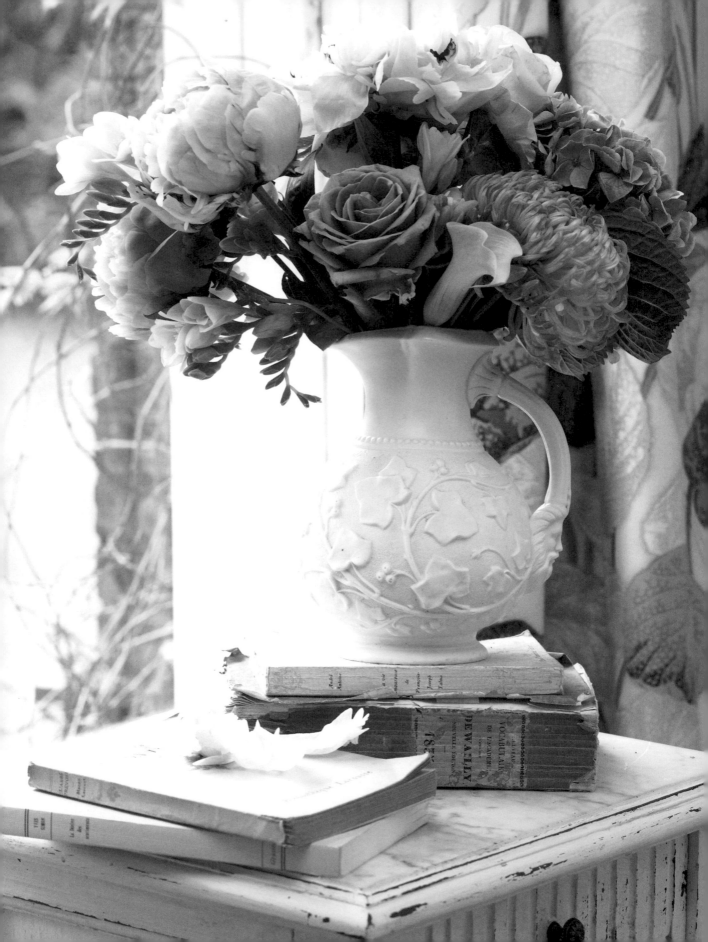

Introduction

Ready to start living a more holistic life in tune with natural rhythms? Then dive right in. The best way to begin is to turn to the season that you are living through now. Working with the energy of each season in turn will mean that the ideas should seem easy to follow, the advice natural and the treatments alluring. But if you want to get the best from the book, or have a particular issue you need to clear up right away, take a moment to read this introduction. Here you begin to get into the flow…

Creating your at-home spa

Throughout this book you will find instructions for at-home spa treatments. These therapeutic treatments will nurture your body, but the wonderful bonus is that they will also relax your mind. The power of ritual soothes and calms. The sense of actually setting time aside to pamper yourself is restorative in itself. We believe that by lavishing extra attention on your body, you'll become more aware of the wonder of 'the skin you're in'. You'll grow in self-confidence and self-acceptance.

And, of course, you will look your absolute best, too.

The soothing effect will be heightened if you take the time to clear a shelf in your bathroom or bedroom to store your spa necessities. These should be used by you alone; they should be dedicated to your pleasure. You don't have to spend a lot of money but keeping a few basics to hand, rather than having to search around for them, means that you will be more likely to turn to this book and the ideas within it (and thus relax and restore yourself) far more often.

The Champneys' collection of skincare, bath and body products is another way, besides this book, that we make the Champneys' experience available to everyone. The collection contains all that you need to create an atmosphere of luxury and indulgence at home. You can explore the collection at www.champneys.com, and we give some recommendations here of 'hero' products that are good investments for your at-home spa. But you can also substitute your own favourite products, customise them or even make your own scrubs, soaks and body oils – we show you how overleaf.

Another hint: change the products or scent with the seasons. Doing this will underline to you the qualities of each season – and it also makes sense on an intuitive level. Some aromatherapy oils speak more of one season than another but don't let this inhibit you from using your intuition when reaching for a scent. Lavender is naturally associated with summer but it will help relax you at any time of year. (If you're pregnant, restrict yourself to lavender.)

For spring: choose an energising fragrance, citrus-based, or a detoxing, oceanic one.

- Champneys' keynote ranges: the Aqua Therapy range or the Citrus Glow range.

Key aromatherapy oils:

- Bergamot – uplifting, fights stress-induced exhaustion.
- Mandarin – calms and rejuvenates.
    - Peppermint – invigorating, refreshing.
    - Grapefruit – restores emotional equilibrium, banishes moodiness, anger and stress

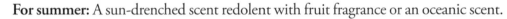

For summer: A sun-drenched scent redolent with fruit fragrance or an oceanic scent.

- Champneys' keynote ranges: the Exotic range which has mango, uplifting palmarosa and sensual ylang-ylang, or the Aqua Therapy range.

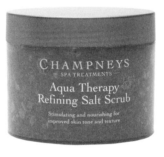

Create your own with:

- May chang – uplifting, sparkling.
- Ylang-ylang – puts you in touch with your spiritual side, boosts self-esteem.
- Jasmine – sensual, sweet, soothing.
- Neroli – melts away anxiety, lifts the spirits.

For autumn: A nourishing, balancing scent.

- Champneys' keynote range: the Rose range, fragrant with rose damascene.
  Create your own with:

- Rose – calms, brings emotional balance, diminishes grief.

- Rosemary – invigorating, muscle relaxer.

    - Geranium – balancing, cheering, gives back a sense of control.

        - Juniper – strengthening, purifying, refreshing.

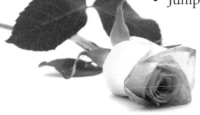

For winter: A comforting, soothing scent.

- Champneys' keynote range: the Oriental range, with vanilla and sandalwood.
  Create your own with:

- Sandalwood – sensual.

- Patchouli – blows away the blues and stress.

- Chamomile – comforting and deeply relaxing.

    - Frankincense – calms the mind, soothes the spirit, helps you reach
      a meditative state, inspiring.

You'll also need some essential equipment and general products:

  - A loofah or exfoliating mitts and an exfoliating scrub.

  - A selection of invigorating shower gels and relaxing bath soaks.

- An enriching body lotion to moisturise your skin after treatment.

You will benefit from:

- A heavy-duty body butter, too, for times when your skin needs intensive
moisturising.

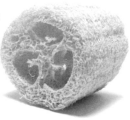

- A massager or you could buy a wooden roller so you can apply pressure
in hard-to-reach areas.

- A natural bristle body brush for skin brushing before a treatment, or dry textured mitts.
- A facial exfoliater and/or exfoliating brush.

These extras are not essential, but they will really help:
- A pair of cotton gloves for intensive hand moisturising.
- A pair of soft night socks for intensive foot moisturising.
- A scented candle or aromatherapy diffuser.
- An enveloping towelling robe.

Build a collection of essential oils and you have at your fingertips an elegant way to transform your mood and the means of creating your own treatments for adding to the bath, moisturising and treating the skin, or adding to sugar scrubs.

Scrub recipe
Add 10 drops of essential oil to 10 ml of base oil. Take four large handfuls of caster sugar and mix into a paste with the oils.

Soak recipe
Add 10 drops of your chosen aromatherapy oil to a cup of Epsom salt (from the chemists) and dissolve in a warm bath. Sip a glass of water throughout, and avoid salts if you have a circulatory disease.

Body oil recipe
Take 100 ml of base oil (sweet almond, wheatgerm, jojoba or a combination) and add 20–40 drops of essential oil, depending on your preferences. If there is any left, keep it in a dark glass bottle with a tight stopper, which you can buy from a health food shop.

Classic combinations:
- To revive you: grapefruit, rosemary, bergamot.
- To restore you: frankincense, rose, geranium.
- To calm you: mandarin, rose, juniper or lavender.

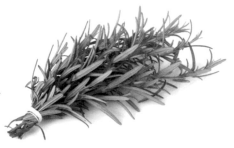

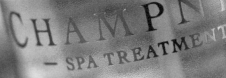

CHAMPNEYS
— SPA TREATMENTS —

Perfect Sleep
Pillow Mist

Hero products

- Champneys Exotic Bubble Float – turns any bath into a spa experience, with ylang-ylang, mango and palmarosa.

- Champneys Perfect Sleep Pillow Mist contains a pure essential oil blend of balancing mandarin, comforting chamomile and relaxing lavender.

- Champneys Pure Relaxation Massage Oil contains olive-derived squalane, a key component of the skin's own natural moisturising system, giving it a very skin-friendly formula. The oil is a blend of lavender, to relax and balance the whole body, mandarin to uplift and chamomile to comfort.

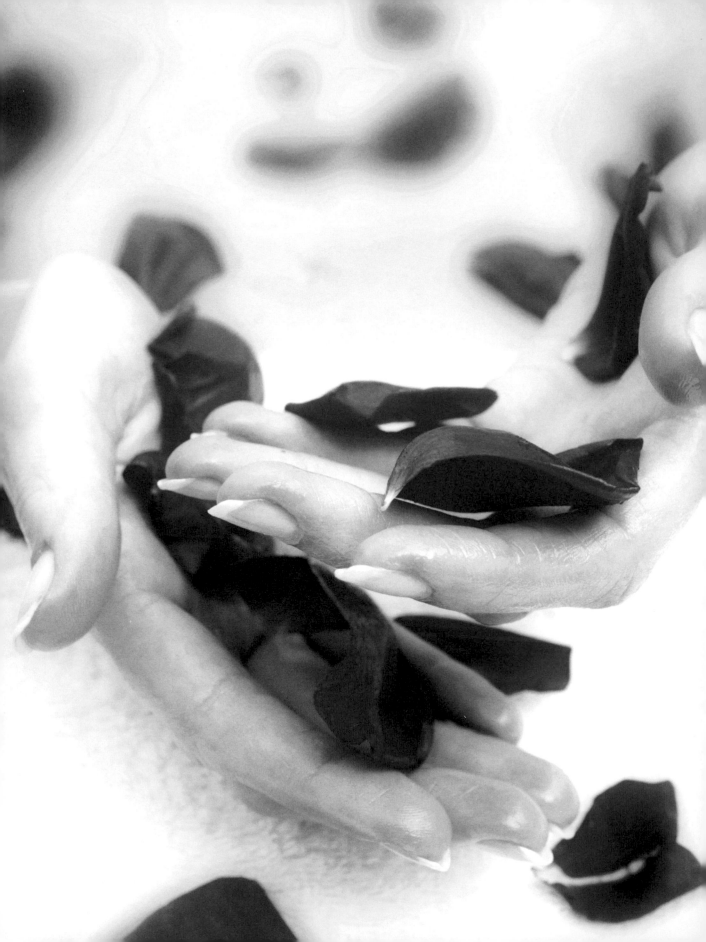

But where are you right now?

Travel through the year with us and you'll naturally address each aspect of your health and well-being at the time when it will be easiest to make changes. But what if you are feeling tired, run down and fed up and want to start addressing the root causes immediately? Take the following quiz which will help you play detective and navigate your way instantly to the most important part of the book for you right now.

You are feeling tired, rundown and lacking in energy. Yes?

Answer these questions: Yes No

1. Are you active, 'on the go' for at least an hour a day?   ☐   ☐

2. Do you exercise five days a week for at least half an hour a day?   ☐   ☐

3. Do you watch less than an hour of TV a day?   ☐   ☐

4. Do you have good posture?   ☐   ☐

5. Do you spend more hours moving around than seated?   ☐   ☐

Answering 'no' to just one of these shows something that could be affecting your energy levels.

Energy production depends on some specific physiological reactions – for instance, enough oxygen has to reach your cells where it is needed to metabolise glucose, your body's fuel. Smoking is terrible for energy levels because it inhibits oxygen flow. Bad posture doesn't help either.

It's been shown that you use minutely more calories lying on the couch doing nothing than lying on the couch watching TV, presumably because when you're doing nothing at least your brain is working; when you're watching TV, it's not (or not so much). On the other hand, 'active relaxation' – such as walking, yoga and other forms of exercise – actually helps energise you rather than tire you out. Turn to page 41 for some gentle ideas on boosting energy quickly.

You feel listless, have skin or gut problems and are frequently run down. Yes?

Answer these questions: Yes No

   1. Do you always eat breakfast? ☐ ☐

   2. Do you always eat lunch? ☐ ☐

   3. Do you eat three meals a day and occasional snacks? ☐ ☐

   4. Do you eat at least five fruit and vegetable portions a day? ☐ ☐

   5. Do you eat wholegrains (brown pasta, bread, rice) in preference to white? ☐ ☐

   6. Do you drink two or fewer cups of tea or coffee per day? ☐ ☐

   7. Do you spread your calories throughout the day, concentrating most ☐ ☐
      in the morning and lunch?

Score one for each 'yes'. Even one 'no' could mean your diet is letting you down and leading to lack of energy and poor concentration. Answer 'no' to most questions and it could be affecting your immune system. If you scored five or fewer, turn to page 20 for some easy ideas to power up your nutrition. To have enough energy you need enough good-quality food providing your cells with energy. You also need to eat regularly enough for your energy production to remain strong and constant. Eat every three hours – that's healthier than relying on caffeine to keep you going.

You are exhausted and 'wired'. Yes?

Answer these questions: Yes No

   1. Do you get fewer than seven or eight hours of good quality sleep most nights? ☐ ☐

   2. Do you have young children who sometimes wake up during the night? ☐ ☐

   3. Do you often wake during the night, even if you get back to sleep easily? ☐ ☐

   4. Do you feel tired in the morning even after a normal night's sleep? ☐ ☐

   5. Do you feel exhausted in the afternoon? ☐ ☐

If you answered 'yes' to two or more questions, it's a sign that your sleep levels are affecting your well-being. Be ruthless in seeking out the causes. According to the American Psychological Association, stress is the number one cause of middle-of-the-night waking and insomnia. If you know something is keeping you awake at night, the only solution is to keep on pressing until you find a solution. Turn to page 207 for the Champneys 'sleep deep' plan. By the way, at somewhere between six to nine months, little children can be helped to settle through the night. If your children are older but still disturbing your sleep, it might be worth seeking professional help from a children's sleep clinic.

You are exhausted and 'wired', but you are getting seven to eight hours of good quality sleep. Yes?

Answer these questions:

	Yes	No
1. Do you frequently take work home at weekends?	☐	☐
2. Do you often get angry with shop assistants, other drivers or your family for being too slow?	☐	☐
3. Do you feel depressed when you think of your working life?	☐	☐
4. Do you have less than an hour a day to yourself to relax and recharge?	☐	☐
5. Do you have a drink most evenings purely to unwind after a hard day?	☐	☐
6. When you come home, do you go immediately into domestic chores?	☐	☐
7. Do you sometimes not take all your annual holiday leave?	☐	☐
8. Do you feel you spend too little quality time with your family and friends?	☐	☐

Score one for each 'yes'. If you score three or more, your work–life balance is out of kilter. The 90:120 rule should help. Plan your working day in 120-minute blocks which is the absolute longest most people can maintain focus, according to US research. After 90 minutes stop, take a couple of minutes break and when you return to work do another sort of task until you've reached the 120-minute mark. After two hours, plan what you'll do for the next 120-minute block. This should improve productivity. For more tips on achieving a work–life balance that works for you, turn to page 213.

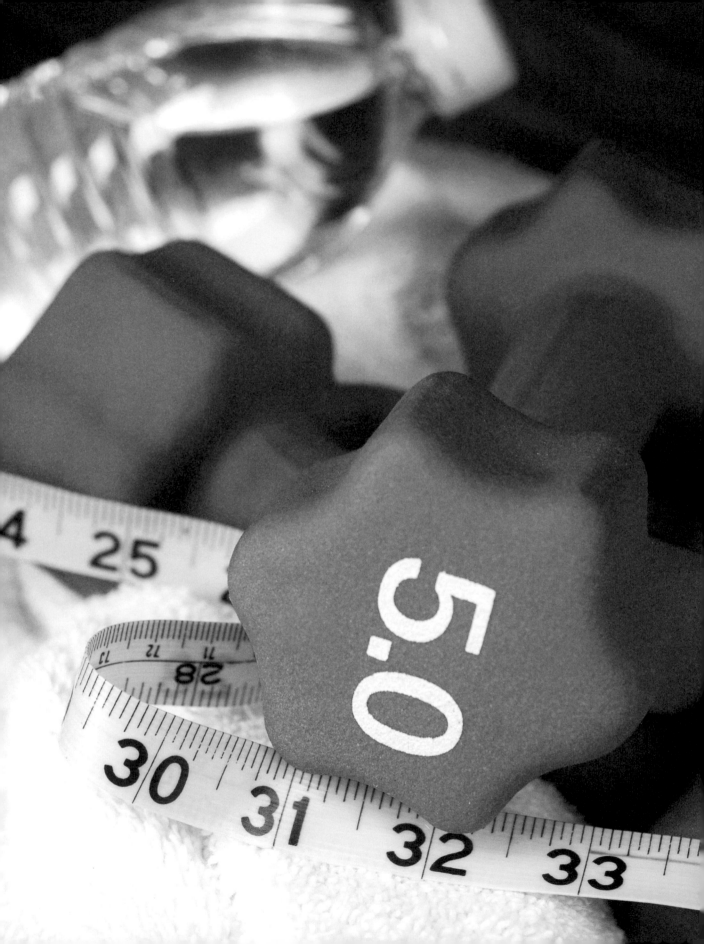

Sensible precautions

It is important to be sensible about starting a new regime, and this is particularly true with exercise. Here are some things you should consider before starting out and which you should bear in mind as you exercise:

- Before starting to work out, make sure you get a full physical from your doctor and a letter stating that it is OK for you to do physical activity. Many gyms will require this before letting you start.

- If you're a beginner, it's a good idea to seek the advice of a fitness trainer – whether it's a personal trainer or a trainer at your gym – to be sure your form is safe and correct.

- Wear suitable clothing and footwear for the activity that you choose to do.

- Drinking lots of water is important. When you exercise, your body loses plenty of water as you sweat so it's important to rehydrate yourself. Water will also help cleanse your body and it's good for your skin too.

- It is also important to make sure you stretch each time – both before and after your exercise. If you suffer from heart disease or have a history of high blood pressure consult your doctor before exercising. Stop exercising immediately if you experience any pain. If you suffer from arthritis in certain joints avoid these areas when they are inflamed and painful.

Now join us travelling through a Champneys' year. Prepare to feel relaxed, revived and restored…

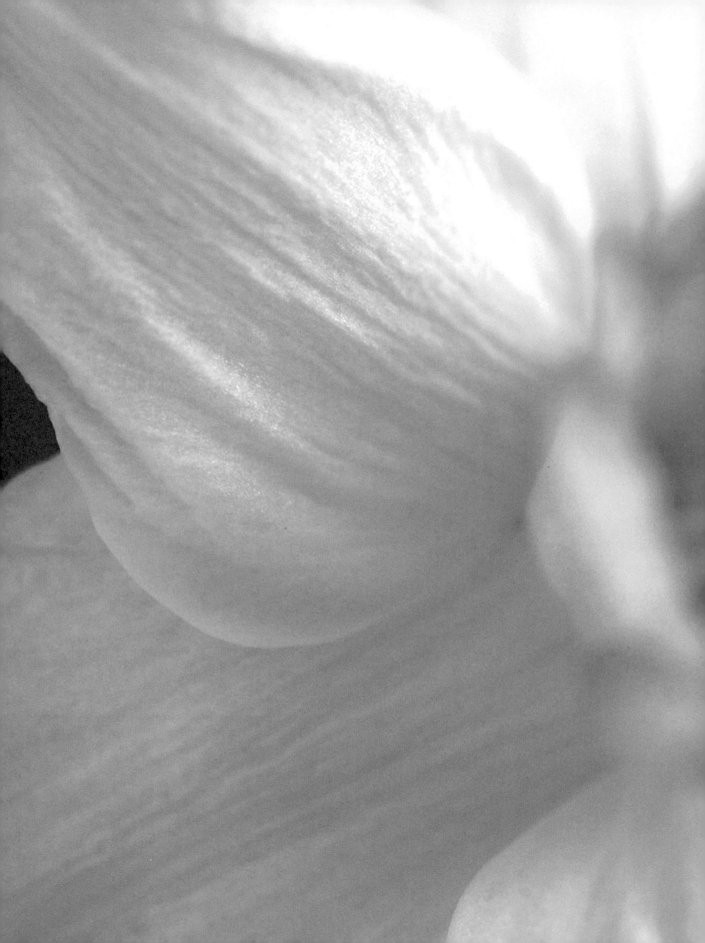

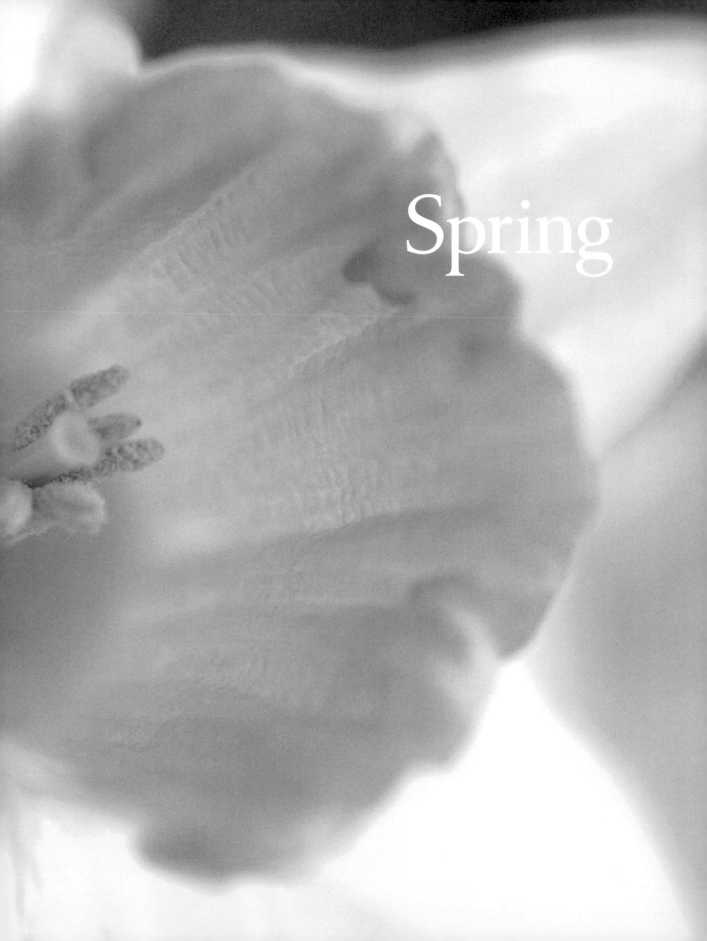

Spring

Five ways to celebrate spring

- Throw open the window every chance you get. Become conscious of your breath. Take a minute during the day to breath in deeply; what can you smell? Spring has its own distinct scent. Now become conscious of where you are holding tension in your body and breathe it out. This is the speediest stress-buster ever.

- Start taking a multi-vitamin and mineral if you are not already doing so. It will support your nutritional goals.

- Clear out... a room, the garage, a drawer, your handbag. Shedding unwanted clutter will free your mind.

- Book a massage. Loosen the tension built up throughout the winter. Get reacquainted with your body again after the big cover-up of winter.

- Love your mum, cherish your daughter. Mothers' day falls in spring. This is the time to celebrate the important women in your life. Why not book a day together at a spa, or treat each other to some of the treatments in this book?

Everything seems possible…

March is a great month to…

indulge in some new bed linen and spend a morning in bed (or a whole day) lounging and dozing. The spring equinox falls in March and the clocks change this month. This can upset our sleep patterns. Make sure you catch up.

April is a great month to…

buy a raincoat. This is such a magical month, don't be put off from enjoying nature by the April showers (Champneys supply waterproofs in every bedroom). Walking in the soft spring rain is a tonic in itself.

May is a great month to…

follow Champneys' three-day 'Be Rejuvenated' programme. There are two bank holidays this month – can you devote one three-day holiday to you?

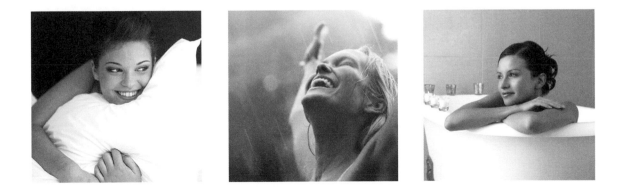

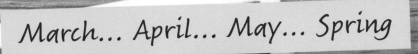
March... April... May... Spring

Energise – take it outside
and tune into nature...

New beginnings – spring is the season of
birth and renewal... nodding daffodils, the
sweet smell of hyacinths, bursts of yellow,
pink and creamy white in the hedges and
garden, and carpets of bluebells in dappled
sunlight.

Purify – be rejuvenated. Shed everything
that is holding you back ... Cleanse from
the inside out with a gentle approach to
detoxing.

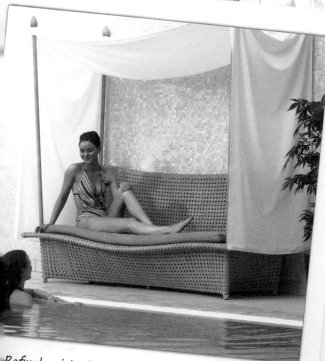

Discover — a new, laid-back attitude to food... Polish skin, banish puffiness and emerge a radiant version of yourself this spring. Blossom on trees, birdsong and lighter nights will lift your mood as well as your energy levels and make it easy to adopt changes that will support and nourish your long-term health.

Fresh start... yours begins here.

Refresh with deeply invigorating treatments and instant beautifiers...

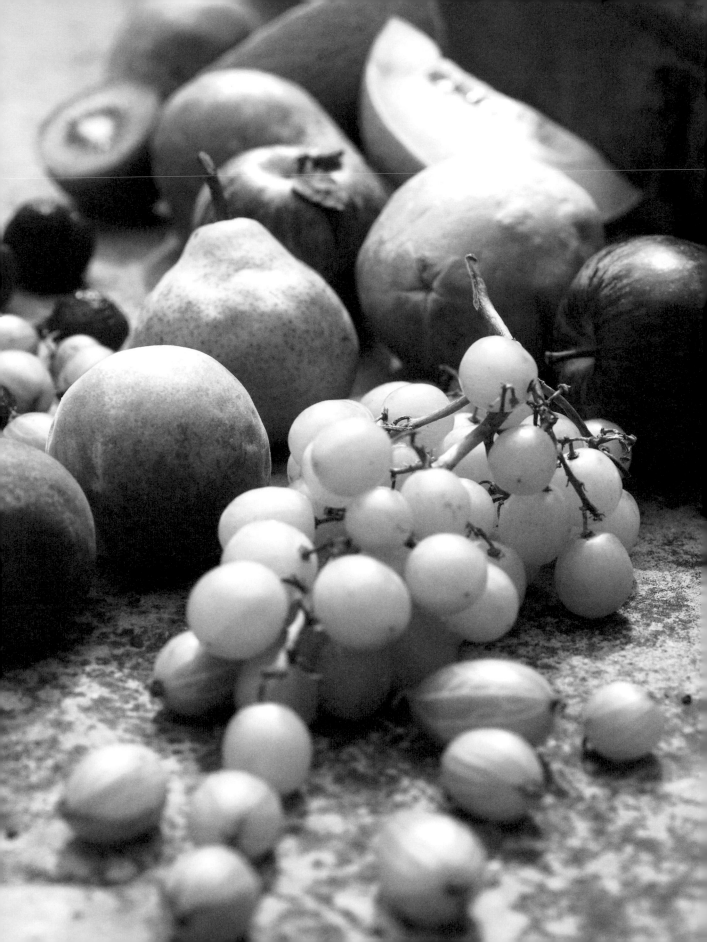

Eat

Easy does it... Every morning is a brand new opportunity to improve your health, well-being and mood. One of the most straightforward ways of doing that is by eating the sort of food that supports and nourishes you. Spring is the perfect season to rethink your relationship with food if you're not eating as well as you'd like. As the days warm and lengthen, we are naturally drawn to less heavy food. This is the time – not the middle of winter – when it's easy to resolve to eat well.

Everyone knows why it's important. Eating healthily supplies you with the energy you need to get through your day effortlessly and calmly. It provides you with the nutrients that will protect your long-term health and repair damage done by stress and pollution. It keeps you looking fabulous today, and for years to come, by age-proofing your body.

At Champneys when it comes to food, we steer away from fads and fallacies. We don't count calories. Instead we help our guests make healthy choices based on the latest scientific findings about optimum nutrition and health.

With this approach, food, rather than being the enemy, becomes an ever-present source of delight and reassurance. Every meal becomes a chance to choose food that not only tastes delicious but will also nourish your body and ensure long-term health. To get to this point, don't think of cutting out the (unhealthy) foods you enjoy, but instead think of 'adding in' the delicious, nutritious foods that are going to help you look and feel terrific. Concentrate on 'adding in' goodness and you find your desire for less healthy food dissipates.

Make it easy on yourself

You could decide to embark on a weight-reducing diet right now, but you have just emerged from winter's hibernation, and this is the time to fortify and cleanse your body rather than put it under too much pressure.

Eating healthily doesn't have to be a chore – take it easy, one simple step at a time. Every week make one change to your diet. Devise your own plan or follow our suggestions; look at the spring-themed recipes on pages 31–38 for inspiration.

It can be very difficult to change the way we eat, partly because our relationship with food is often bound up with habits that we think are essential to our happiness. We feel we need to have two coffees before we can function, must head for that night in the pub to unwind, and don't even question the ice-cream blow-out that marks every fight with a partner. But by gradually integrating new habits we can move elegantly into a new way of eating, shedding our old habits without even noticing. We 'add in' healthy food to the extent that we have no room left for the unhealthy, except very occasionally – just as it should be!

Revolutionise the way you eat – one step at a time!

After twelve weeks of 'adding in' healthy food to your existing diet, you will have transformed your eating habits – without much effort. Use our plan here, or devise your own…

• **Week 1.** Resolve to eat a good breakfast every morning. Your metabolic rate slows down overnight and without eating breakfast you can stay on this lower rate until lunchtime. It's been estimated that this alone can result in a 1 kilo weight gain every year – which might explain why regular breakfast eaters weigh, on average, 4 kilos less than non-breakfast eaters. For those who dislike eating breakfast, try smoothies. (Turn to page 32) for some inspiration.) A perfect breakfast includes complex carbohydrates, protein and fruit or vegetables.

• **Week 2.** Eat at least one portion of fruit or vegetables at every meal and snack on it twice a day. You will then be hitting the (bare minimum) recommendation of five portions a day. Most experts would recommend getting around eight to ten. So if you can make it two portions each meal – even better!

• **Week 3.** Drink a glass of water with every meal and when you go to the loo. The reputable Mayo Institute in the US has recognised lack of water as a prime reason for energy dips. There is always a debate whether we really need 1.5 litres of water a day – but it's a no-brainer. Fluid is essential to feeling well and since water is almost unique in being a fluid with no downside – no caffeine, calories, alcohol, sugar – surely it becomes the perfect choice.

• **Week 4.** Aim for at least one portion of wholegrains, beans or lentils a day. Your eventual target should be three a day so try, by the end of the week, to be eating one at each meal. One cup of cooked oats, half a cup of wholegrain pasta or rice, quinoa, beans or pulses or half a slice of wholegrain bread at each meal will help your energy levels – and contribute to your daily fibre intake which is important for protecting you against heart disease and cancer.

• **Week 5.** Aim for at least one portion of lower fat dairy products in a day like a small tub of natural yoghurt or 40g of goat's cheese (about the size of your thumb).

• **Week 6.** Eat a bowl of salad leaves a day – rocket, lettuce, basil, parsley, watercress – as a first course before lunch or dinner. Grate a little carrot or apple over your leaves or add some home-made vinaigrette, balsamic vinegar or olive oil. (Research shows that eating a small salad before meals contributes to weight loss.)

• **Week 7.** Cut your salt intake by half, both in cooking and at the table. From that point, continuing to reduce it gradually will wean you off salt – and you will begin to enjoy the taste of food without it.

• **Week 8.** Swap one of your regular cups of caffeinated drink for a healthier brew. Decaf is better but why not go for a cup of tea that positively boosts health? Green tea appears to speed up metabolism and protects you against Alzheimer's; redbush (or Rooibus) tea is caffeine-free and loaded with antioxidants.

• **Week 9.** Aim for one portion of soya products a day – half a cup of beans, a small tub of plain soya yoghurt, a portion of tofu the size of a deck and a half of cards or 225ml of soya milk. Two portions a day have been shown to reduce the risk of heart disease.

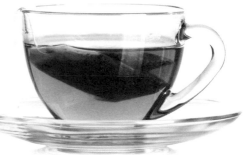

• **Week 10.** Make your alcoholic intake 'mindful'. Don't just throw alcohol back because it's there; think 'do I really want this?' If you do drink alcohol, make it a special occasion, and really savour both the taste and the occasion. And if you're actually not that bothered, order a soft drink instead. It's true that one or two small glasses of wine a day help protect against heart disease – but only in men and post-menopausal women. In women before the menopause, there are no added benefits to the heart and research shows even one drink a day can raise the risk of breast cancer. Limit alcohol intake to moderate levels (fourteen units a week for women, twenty-one for men) but don't drink mindlessly.

• **Week 11.** Find a new way to include fish in your diet every day. Does your local sandwich bar serve a shrimp salad? Could you take a tinned salmon sandwich to work for lunch? Shredded smoked mackerel fillets on toast make a tasty breakfast. And, of course, this is the perfect week to try some of Champneys' fish recipes. The challenge of choosing fish every day should open your eyes to how easy it is to get the recommended two to three servings a week from now on.

• **Week 12.** Snack on a handful of nuts a day – Around 25g a day protects your heart, and pistachios, cashews, almonds, walnuts and pecans make a great mid-afternoon snack as they cut hunger pangs.

'Nuts are a great fast food – and a really healthy choice for a snack. What's more, research shows that nuts – in moderation (about a small handful a day) – can help keep you slim.'

– AILSA HIGGINS, CHAMPNEYS' NUTRITIONIST

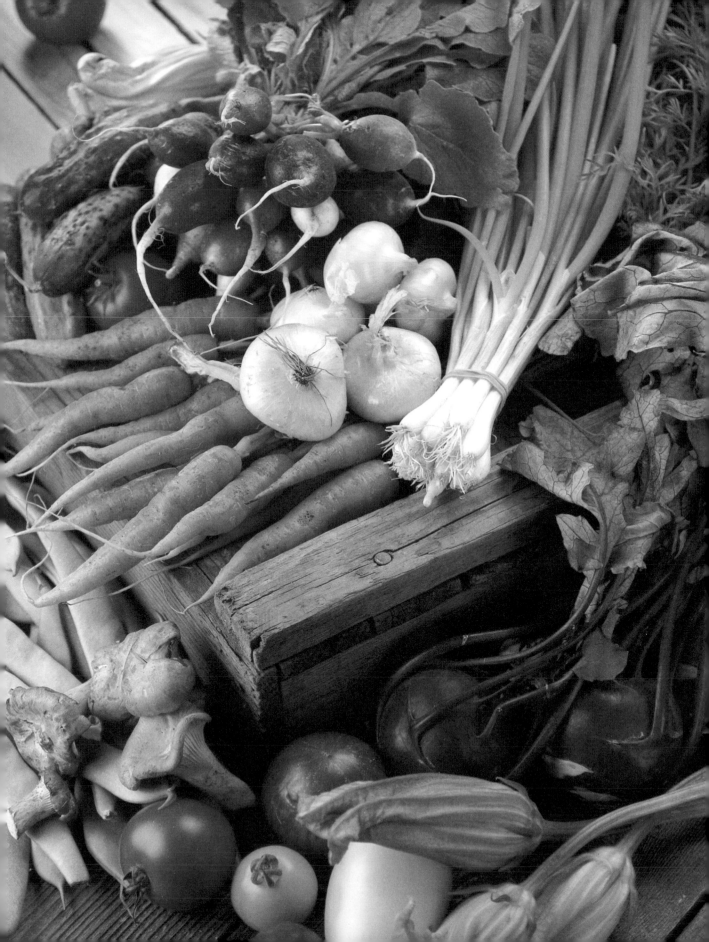

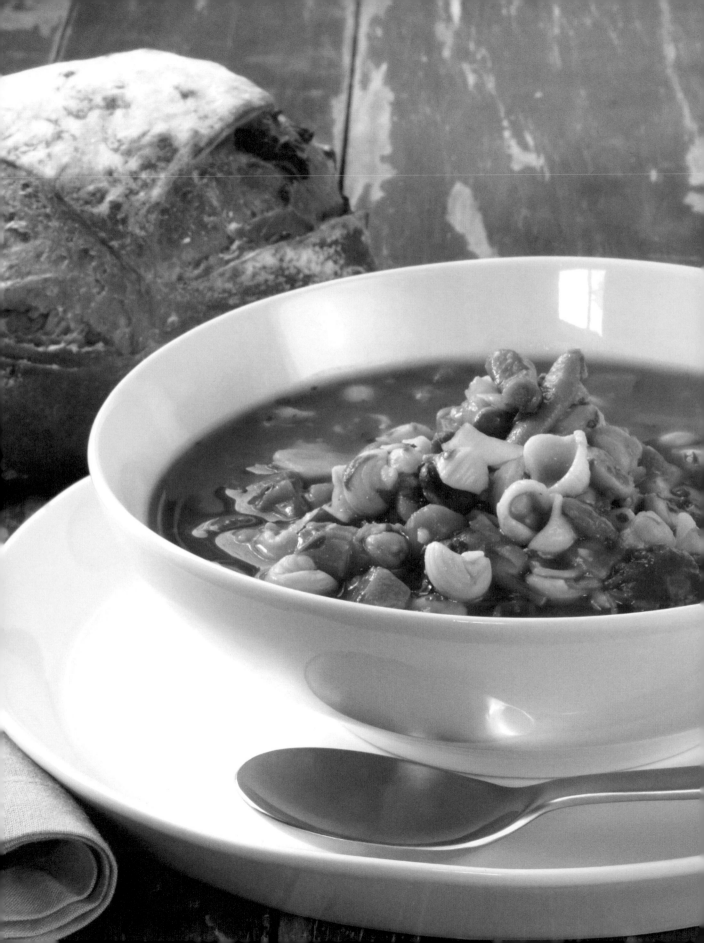

So what do you feel like eating today?

A comforting bowl of hearty vegetable soup? A delicious salad brimming with crunch and colour? A delicately flavoured piece of grilled fish? A glass of aromatic wine? Your choice. Your pleasure. Your future health – on a plate.

When making your decision, bear in mind these three fundamentals of truly healthy eating:

• **Moderation.** Do not overload your stomach. In the East, a rule of thumb is that a meal should in total be the equivalent of one moderate bowlful. Eat slowly and savour each mouthful. After a couple of weeks, you will find that you don't want more than a bowlful of food at any one time.

• **Balance.** The three main food groups (protein, carbohydrate, fat) should all be represented in the right proportion. We make it easy for our guests with the Champneys' plate (see page 89) but as a rule of thumb, when putting together a meal, remember **LATE:**

Load up with vegetables and fruit. Most of your meal should be plant-based, and fill half your plate with non-starchy vegetables.

Add in protein. A little protein – a piece the size and thickness of your palm – at every meal gives you energy and keeps hunger at bay.

Two tablespoons of wholegrain carbohydrates, starchy vegetables, beans or pulses keep you calm and happy, and stop cravings for unhealthy foods.

Extras. A small amount of healthy fats is essential for health.

• **Variety.** To achieve the 'well-balanced' diet that we are always hearing about we should be choosing from between sixty to seventy different foodstuffs. It's been estimated that the average person eats only around twenty. Without a wide variety of foods we can't get all the vitamins and trace minerals we need for optimum health. Make it a rule of thumb to try a new food or a seasonal one every week.

Makeover your shop

Swap	For
Sweets, biscuits, cakes The odd treat is fine but these should not be part of your routine shop as they disrupt your body's chemistry and add nutritionally empty calories.	**Fruit, mostly fresh, a little dried** Naturally sweet, thanks to the sugars they contain, but loaded with antioxidants that mop up the 'free radicals' (the by-products of biological pathways in your body that cause disease if not eliminated).
White pasta, rice, bread and sugary cereals These supply energy but have relatively little nutritional value, and cereals and bread will probably have sugar and salt added.	**Wholemeal and wholegrain products, beans and pulses** Wholegrain bread, pasta and rice; porridge; barley; quinoa; chick peas; lentils – beans and pulses of all sorts are higher in nutrients and fibre. They are also great at bulking out meals. Try a lentil or bean salad instead of a pile of pasta and you'll be powering up the nutritional value of your meal.
Red meat and meat products such as sausages, bacon and burgers Cutting down on red meat (aim to eat it no more than once or twice a week) will cut saturated fat and your risk of developing diseases such as heart disease and bowel cancer.	**More fish (especially oily fish), beans and pulses** Aim to eat fish two to three times a week and oily fish (such as mackerel, herring, salmon or fresh tuna) twice a week. Organic lean meat and game, is a good source of protein, too, but choosing vegetarian and fish recipes for the majority of your week's meals will improve your long-term health.
Processed foods Anything not in its natural state will have its nutrients ripped out and additives, salt and sugar added. This includes most of our popular snacks and 'treats'.	**Vegetables, salads, nuts and seeds** A handful of nuts is filling and good for your heart. Nibbling on thinly sliced and diced raw vegetables fills you up, and a crunchy salad is way more satisfying than a bag of crisps.
Caffeinated drinks These drinks give you energy but they also cause energy slumps.	**Water and herbal teas** These will give you energy and a sense of control rather than contributing to your stress levels.
Some butter and most margarines Cut out all those spreads with hydrogenated or partially hydrogenated fat in the listed ingredients. A little butter is fine, but keep intake low because it's also high in the saturated fat that is bad for the heart.	**Healthy oils such as olive or rapeseed** These are high in the healthy fatty acids that protect your heart, and provide antioxidants. Try dipping bread into a little oil rather than slathering on butter at every meal, or blend butter with oils to make your own spread which confers health benefits as well as taste.

Your basket at a glance

Loads of fruits and vegetables.

Lean meat, fish (some of it oily).

Tins of beans and pulses.

Eggs, cheese, low-fat milk, soya milk or yoghurts.

Healthy oils, nuts, seeds and olives.

Wholegrain bread, pasta, rice.

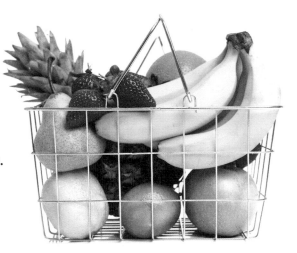

Eating seasonally – choosing foods that are in season – is the buzzword just now. But let's not forget the health benefits of eating unseasonally. These are the foods that should be staples in your trolley, whatever the season.

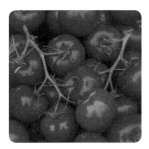

• **Tinned tomatoes.** Studies reveal that people who eat a lot of tomato-based foods are less likely to get cancer. It's the lycopene, which gives the tomato its red colour, that makes it a powerful antioxidant, and it works best when it is cooked. Tinned tomatoes, tomato paste and cooked tomatoes are actually a better choice than fresh. (Try them warmed and on toast for breakfast.)

• **Tinned beans and pulses.** Beans or pulses are full of polyphenols, an important antioxidant. Eating beans four times a week could cut your risk of heart disease by 22%. They're also a great source of fibre which helps to reduce 'bad' cholesterol and raise 'good' cholesterol. Keeping tinned beans and pulses to hand means you can add them easily to soups, casseroles and salads.

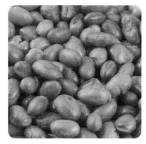

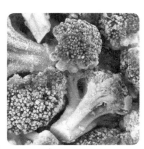

• **Frozen vegetables.** Most frozen produce is frozen immediately after harvest so nutrient concentration is higher than in fresh veg. Steaming maintains this high concentration; boiling for prolonged periods reduces it.

• **Frozen fruit.** Berries – blackberries, blackcurrants, redcurrants, cranberries, strawberries – are rich in anthocyanins, antioxidants that work with vitamin C. They reverse the ageing of the brain and reduce blood pressure. Add them to a smoothie, yoghurt or porridge.

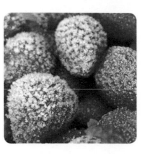

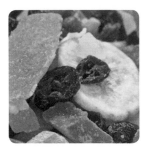

• **Dried fruits.** These are all good at fighting disease though contain higher sugar levels than fresh fruit. Organic is best – pesticides can be concentrated in dried fruit. Include in moderation in salads or cereal or take as a snack when going for a long walk.

• **Nut butter.** This may lower your heart disease risk by 21%. Look for brands which are lower in salt and sugar, and are without hydrogenated (trans) fats. Spread it on wholegrain toast instead of butter or on apple slices for a quick snack.

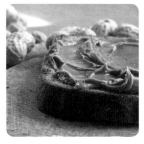

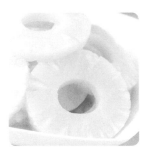

• **Canned pineapple.** Pineapple is not only rich in Vitamin C but also contains bromelain, an enzyme with useful properties including support of digestive function and reduction of blood stickiness (important for reducing the risk of arterial disease). Choose pineapple canned in juice rather than syrup.

• **Soba noodles.** These Japanese noodles are made from buckwheat, a good source of two cancer-fighting antioxidants, quercetin and rutin. Use them in place of less nutritious egg noodles.

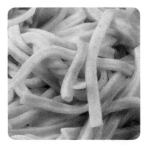

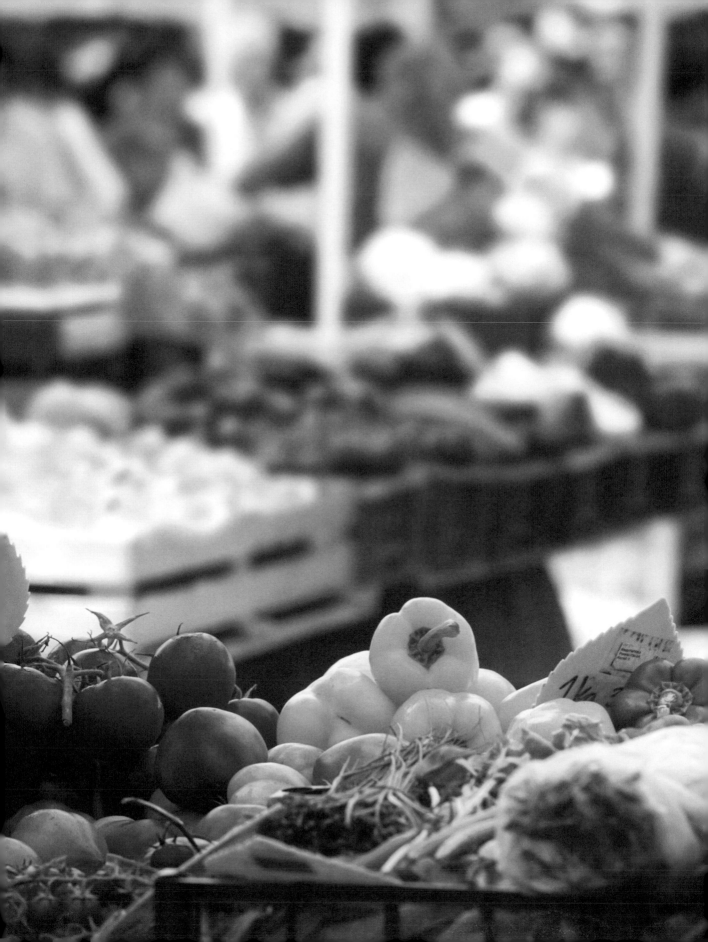

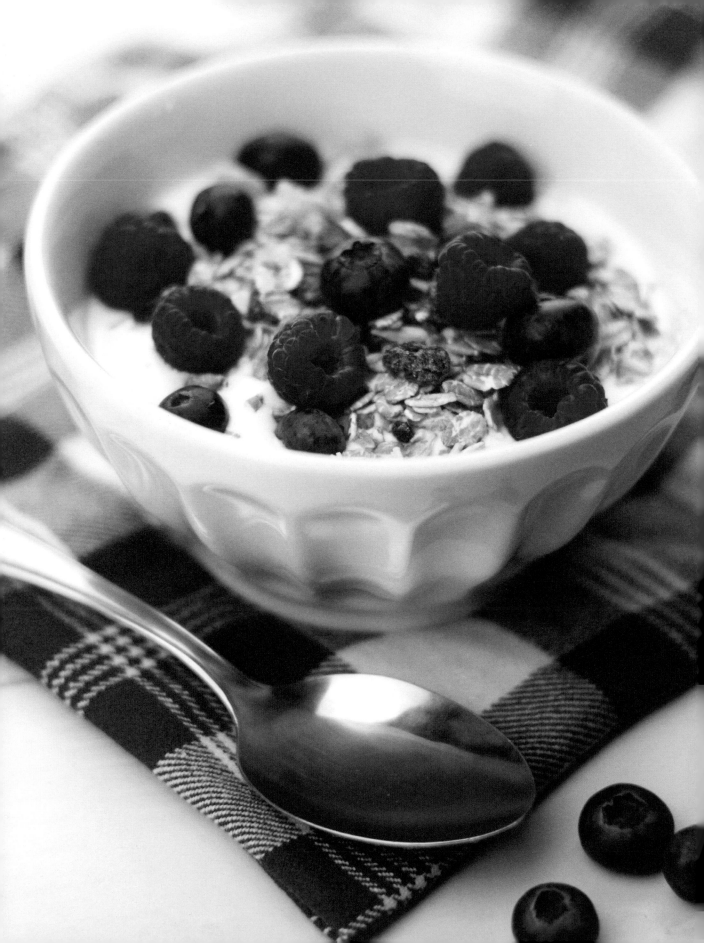

Inspiration to eat well...

Breakfasts

Scrambled eggs, smoked salmon and dill
(serves 2)
3 organic eggs
2 tbsp soya milk
125g smoked Scottish salmon,
    cut into fine strips
1 tsp fresh dill, chopped
1 wholemeal muffin

Break the eggs into a bowl and whisk them with the soya milk. Add the smoked salmon and dill. Pour the mixture into a pan, gently heat it and whisk until the eggs are still ever so slightly runny. Meanwhile, split and toast the muffin, and spread it lightly with butter or a healthy spread. Put half a muffin on each plate, and spoon the cooked scrambled egg carefully onto the muffin. Serve immediately.

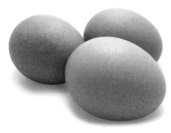

Champneys muesli
(serves 4)
120g porridge oats
25g dried cranberries
25g sultanas
30g chopped hazelnuts
300ml soya milk
30ml orange juice
60ml natural soya yoghurt
Half an apple
Half a pear

Soak all the dry ingredients in the soya milk and leave overnight. Next morning, add the orange juice and soya yoghurt. Peel the fruit and grate it into the muesli; then mix everything together well and serve.

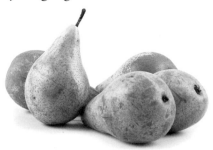

This is a very flexible recipe. You can adapt it by adding different dried fruits or seeds such as pumpkin or sunflower, and might also prefer it with less or no fruit juice.

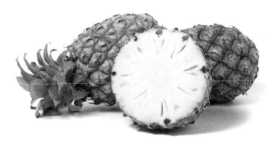

Detox fibre smoothie

(serves 1)

1 mango

200g pineapple, peeled and chopped

2 oranges, peeled and chopped

100g low-fat live natural yoghurt

100ml soya milk

1 tablespoon flaxseed oil

Pinch of ground ginger

Blend all these ingredients together until they are creamy and smooth; serve chilled.

How this smoothie supports your health

- Pineapple, orange and other acidic fruits stimulate the body's natural detoxification systems.

- Live natural yoghurt provides health bacteria to support the digestive system which boosts your natural defences.

- Flaxseed speeds up metabolism

Springs' spring zinger

(serves 1)

1 large pink grapefruit

1 lime

150g frozen raspberries

Juice the ingredients (you may wish to use a citrus press for the grapefruit and lime, and then mix them with the juiced raspberries) and serve immediately.

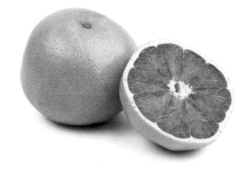

Lunches and main courses

**Celery, apple and walnut salad
with honey and lemon yoghurt**
(serves 1)
75g celery, sliced
Half a green apple, diced
Half a red apple, diced
25g walnut pieces

For the dressing:
25g yoghurt
1 tbsp honey
Grated zest of 2 lemons
Salt and pepper

Put the salad ingredients in a bowl. Whisk the ingredients for the dressing together gently until smooth, and then add the dressing to the bowl with the salad. Mix it well. Put the dressed salad on a plate, garnish it with celery leaves if you like, and serve.

**Haricot beans and avocado salad
with red pepper salsa**
(serves 2)
175g cooked haricot beans
Half an avocado, diced
25g sweetcorn
A handful of fresh coriander, chopped

For the dressing:
2 red peppers, diced
1 onion, diced
2 cloves garlic, chopped
4 plum tomatoes, diced
Juice and zest of 2 limes
100ml white wine vinegar

Mix all the ingredients for the dressing together in a large bowl. Then add the main salad ingredients, stir them together and serve.

Beans and pulses are rich sources of soluble fibre which removes fat from the gut and lowers cholesterol. It also stabilises blood sugar levels and protects against diabetes. Darker beans are particularly rich in protective antioxidant compounds.

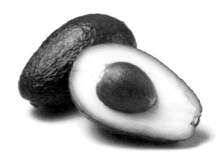

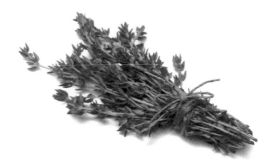

Chargrilled breast of chicken on braised pearl barley with a lemon and thyme yoghurt sauce

(serves 4)

1 onion, finely chopped

1 clove garlic, crushed

Vegetable oil

A small bunch of thyme, chopped

225g pearl barley

600ml chicken stock

   (plus 4 tbsp more for sauce)

salt and pepper

4 x 200g chicken breasts, skinless

150g unsalted butter

150g natural yoghurt

Juice of 1 lemon

Using a heavy-bottomed pan, sweat the onion and garlic in a little vegetable oil until soft and add half the chopped thyme. Then add the pearl barley, cover with chicken stock, season with salt and pepper, and bring to the boil. Cover the pan with a lid, reduce the heat and simmer for 45–60 minutes until soft. Stir the barley while it is cooking to make sure it doesn't catch.

Pre-heat the oven to 180°C / gas mark 4. Chargrill or pan-fry the chicken breasts until they are golden, put them in an ovenproof dish and place them in the oven for 12–15 minutes until they are cooked through (test this by inserting a skewer or fine knife and ensuring that the juices which run out are clear).

Meanwhile, make the sauce. Place the diced butter and about 4 tbsp chicken stock (you may need a little more) in a pan. Bring rapidly to a simmer, whisking frequently. Blitz the sauce with a hand blender and then add the natural yoghurt and lemon juice and blitz it again. Season, and stir in the remaining chopped thyme.

Put a helping of pearl barley in the centre of each plate, cut the chicken pieces in half and place them on top of the pearl barley. Drizzle the sauce around and, if you like, garnish with a sprig of flat parsley.

Chicken can be a calming food. Like turkey, it delivers a steady release of the amino acid tryptophan, which the body can convert to serotonin, a brain chemical that promotes happiness and relaxation. Chicken also provides a dose of stress-essential B vitamins, and zinc.

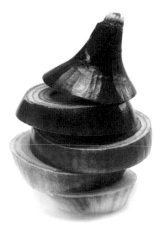

Grilled sea bass with sautéed vegetables and a tomato and onion salsa

(serves 2)

2 sea bass fillets, about 150–175g each

Olive oil

2 carrots, thinly sliced

1 red pepper, deseeded and thinly sliced

2 small leeks, thinly sliced

Salt and pepper

For the salsa:

2 small tomatoes, diced

1 small onion, diced

1 chilli, deseeded and finely chopped

4 tbsp olive oil

2 tsp fresh coriander, chopped

1 clove garlic, chopped

Mix all the salsa ingredients together and season them with salt and pepper. Set it aside. Season the fish fillets and lightly pan fry them, with a little olive oil, skin side first. While the fish is cooking, in a separate pan sauté all the vegetables in a little olive oil until soft and season with a little salt and pepper. Once the fish is ready, put a bed of vegetables on each plate, place the fish on top and drizzle with the salsa.

Sea bass is a source of healthy omega-3 fatty acids and supplies magnesium, too. The salsa contains olive oil which aids the absorption of the magic ingredient in tomatoes, lycopene. It is also beneficial to heart health as it contains healthy monounsaturated fats. Chilli peppers contain capsaicin, a powerful anti-inflammatory which helps joint pains and reduces the risk of diabetes developing.

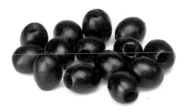

Tapenade-stuffed leg of lamb
(serves 6)
Boned leg of lamb, about 1.5 kg
2 tbsp tapenade (black olive paste)
3 garlic cloves, sliced
2 tbsp rosemary, chopped
Salt and pepper

Preheat the oven to 180ºC / gas mark 4. Oil a roasting pan which is just large enough to hold the lamb, and place a rack in the pan. Now prepare the lamb. Unroll the joint and spread the boned-out side with the tapenade. Roll up the lamb tightly and tie it at 5 cm intervals with kitchen twine. Using a small, sharp knife cut slits 5 cm apart in the top of the joint. Push the garlic slices into the slits. Sprinkle all over with rosemary, salt and pepper.

Roast the lamb for about 1 hour 15 minutes. To check if it's done, insert an instant reading thermometer in the thickest part of the meat. For medium rare, the temperature should be 60–65ºC. Cover the meat loosely with foil and let it rest for at least 30 minutes before slicing it thinly and serving.

Spaghetti with smoked salmon, capers and chilli
(serves 2)
150g spaghetti
1 red onion, chopped
1 red chilli, chopped finely
1 clove garlic, crushed
A handful of chopped flat leaf parsley
Juice of 1 lemon
3 tbsp olive oil
1 tbsp capers
125g smoked salmon, chopped

Cook the spaghetti, following the instructions on the packet. While it is cooking, put the rest of the ingredients in a large bowl and stir them together. Once the pasta is ready, drain well and add it to the bowl. Mix the pasta in well, check the seasoning and serve immediately.

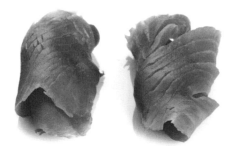

Puddings

Vanilla and orange panna cotta
(serves 5–6)
500ml half-fat cream
75g caster sugar
2 vanilla pods, split in two
Zest of 2 unwaxed oranges
1½ gelatine leaves

Place the cream, sugar, split vanilla pods and orange zest in a saucepan. Bring the mixture to the boil and take the pan off the heat. Meanwhile, soak the gelatine in cold water until soft. Squeeze out the water and whisk the gelatine into the cream mixture. Strain the cream through a sieve into a bowl, and set this over a bowl of ice to cool down. Once the mixture is cold, pour it into moulds (you could also use ramekins) and put it in the fridge for 2 hours or until set.

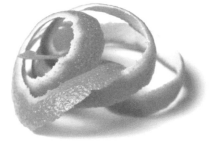

Once they are set, turn the panna cottas out onto the plates. Serve with poached rhubarb, if you like.

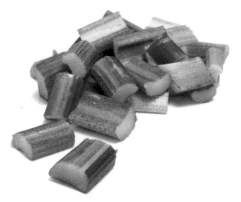

**Gateaux of rice pudding
with a rhubarb compote**
(serves 6)
8 sticks of rhubarb
50g icing sugar
500ml semi-skimmed milk
100g short grain rice
75g caster sugar
25g raisins
1 egg, beaten
100ml crème fraiche

Preheat the oven to 180ºC / gas mark 4. Clean the rhubarb, peeling any tough parts and removing threads, and cut it into large dice. Place these in an ovenproof dish and sprinkle them with the icing sugar. Cover the dish and put it into the oven for 15–20 minutes. Then strain the rhubarb over a colander to collect all the juice and whizz half of it in a blender with the juice you have just collected. Stir the blended rhubarb and juice back into rest of the rhubarb, and leave it to cool. Reduce the oven temperature to 150ºC / gas mark 2.

Boil the milk in a pan and add the rice, caster sugar and raisins. Stir well, and then remove from the heat. Then stir in the egg and pour the mixture into an ovenproof dish. Cover the dish and cook the rice pudding in the low oven for 1½ to 2 hours until cooked – but stir it halfway through cooking. When the rice is ready, remove it from the oven and leave to cool. Once cool, add the crème fraiche and stir. Put the rice pudding into individual bowls, spoon the compote of rhubarb over the top and serve.

In spring, choose these seasonal foods

Rhubarb, radishes, parsley, purple sprouting broccoli, rosemary, spinach, watercress, asparagus, cherries, sea trout, sea bass and spring lamb.

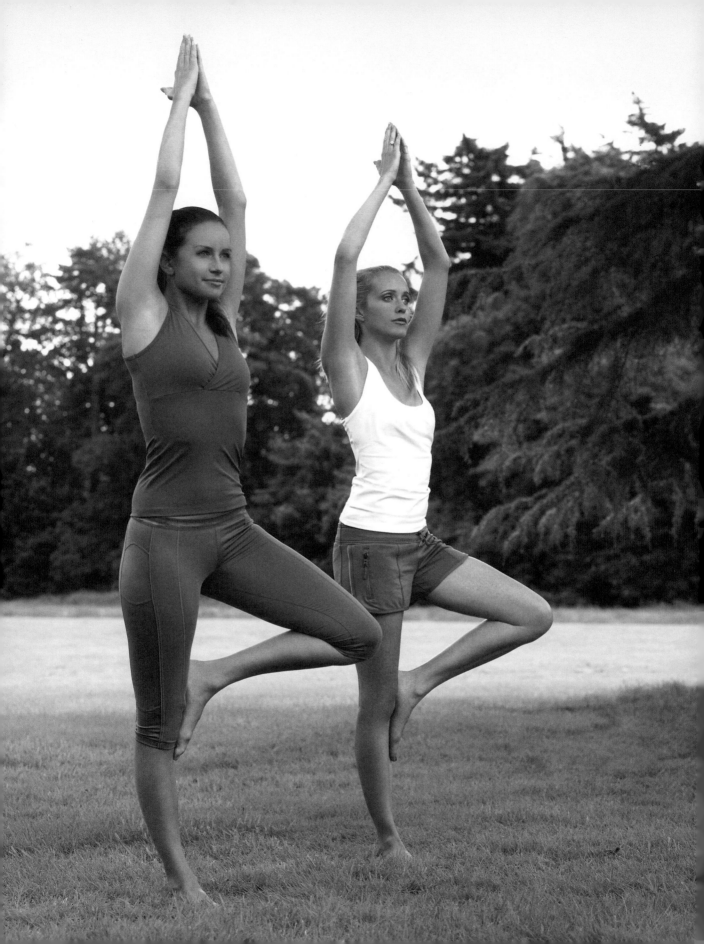

Move

Why you need to move

Do you need a couple of cups of coffee to kickstart your morning? Do you often feel tired and lethargic? Is the only time you feel energised when you're also feeling worried, nervy and tense?

Imagine instead how it would feel to travel through your day, brimming with energy, dealing calmly with everything that life throws at you – in control of your universe. The easiest way to achieve this is through exercise. Regular movement is a necessity. Without it, the only way to be energetic is dosing yourself with stimulants such as caffeine. That means you condemn yourself to swinging between jitteriness and tiredness.

However, by moving your body regularly you trigger off biochemical changes that ensure a constant flow of energy so that you can achieve everything you need to do. Your dependence on artificial stimulants diminishes. Your concentration will improve. Studies show that you will also have a better memory, improved reasoning skills and be more creative.

Learn to walk

If you are already an exercise convert, great. If not, why not start with this easy but extremely effective exercise routine.

Walking gives the benefits of other cardio workouts without the likelihood of injury. It is a great way of easing your way into an exercise regime – all you need are some supportive shoes and, although you can work out on a treadmill at home or in the gym, the terrific thing about walking at this time of the year is that it gets you outside in the fresh air. Spring sunshine will lift your mood. Through exposure to daylight you will replenish your vitamin D levels, diminished through the winter months, and walking outside over changing terrain gives you a better workout.

So grab your shoes and get outside. Walk under the blossom trees, listening to the birdsong, noticing how every week the trees and flowers are blooming more and more. Walking gives you an ideal opportunity to have your feet on the ground and your head in the air – it's a great way to unwind, recharge and energise your batteries.

Warm up, stretch out

This simple warm-up routine is perfect prior to exercise and also a terrific stretching routine to incorporate in a busy day if you've been hunched over a computer or stuck in a stale atmosphere. Master it and you'll have an instant pick-me-up. As you stretch you'll feel your spine lengthening, your chest opening and the blood rushing through your muscles to invigorate and wake you up. These stretches should be carried out before and after walking. Hold each stretch for 10–15 seconds. Ensure that the body is warm prior to stretching – a simple five-minute walk will suffice.

Chest/pectorals
- Stand tall with your feet hip distance apart, and your knees soft.
- Clasp your hands behind your back.
- Keeping your elbows soft, lift your arms up and away behind you whilst squeezing your shoulder blades together.
- Avoid arching your back and keep your abdominals pulled in.

Upper back/trapezius
- Stand with your feet hip distance apart, and your knees soft.
- Clasp your hands in front of you and raise them upwards to shoulder height, whilst rounding your back and lowering your head slightly.
- Imagine you are hugging a beach ball.
- Avoid locking out your elbows.

Front of thigh/quadriceps
- If you need to, use a wall for support. Stand with your feet slightly apart.
- Bend one knee behind you and hold on to the front of your foot.
- Keeping your knees together, gently press your hips forwards, but keeping the heel of your foot away from your bottom.
- Remember to draw your abdominals in, have a slight bend in the supporting leg and stand tall.

Back of thigh/hamstring
- Stand with both feet hip distance apart.
- Place one heel on the floor in front of you, with toes lifted.
- Keeping your back straight, bend the opposite knee and lean forward from the hips, gently pushing your bottom out behind you.
- Place your hands on the supporting knee and keep your head and chest lifted, with abdominals pulled in.

Calf/gastrocnemius

- Take a big step forwards, with your feet parallel and hip distance apart.
- Lean forwards and bend your front knee, keeping it in line with the ankle behind the toes.
- Keep your back heel in contact with the floor at all times.
- Aim for a straight line heel to head, abdominals pulled in.

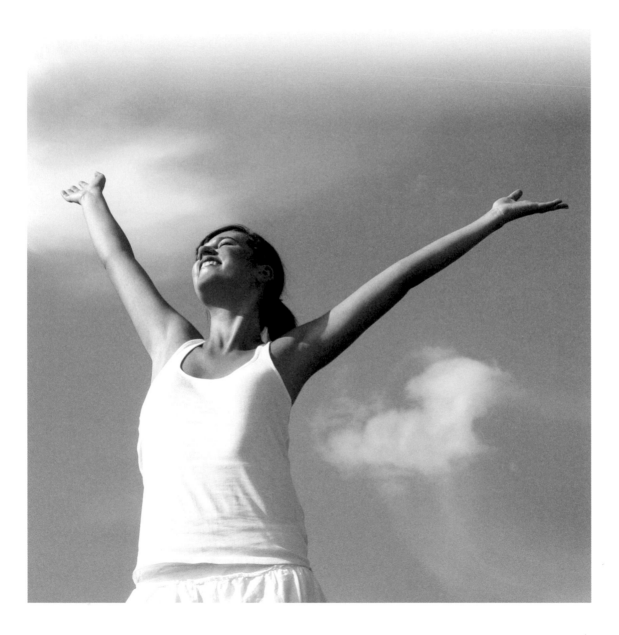

Power into action

Now you're warmed up – start exercising.

- Begin walking at a steady pace.

- Maintain a good posture while you walk. Hold yourself upright, shoulders relaxed and down.

- Select and focus on a spot at eye level and about five metres in front to keep your neck elongated and your chin parallel to the ground. Keep your head up – imagine a string is pulling you up from the top of your head to keep your spine in line.

- Suck it in – contracting your abdominal muscles supports your spine, which in turn helps you keep a good posture. Poor posture can contribute to muscle soreness and stiffness in back, hips and legs.

- Feel your feet as they strike the ground: heel-ball-toe, landing on your heel, rolling through the instep and then pushing off with your toes.

- Swing your arms from the shoulders keeping your elbows at 90 degrees. On the back swing your upper arms should almost be parallel to the ground.

- Nurture your natural stride. To find your natural stride length, experiment by alternating between long and small steps. Somewhere in between you will find a stride that feels right even at a very quick pace, one that does not cause you to bounce.

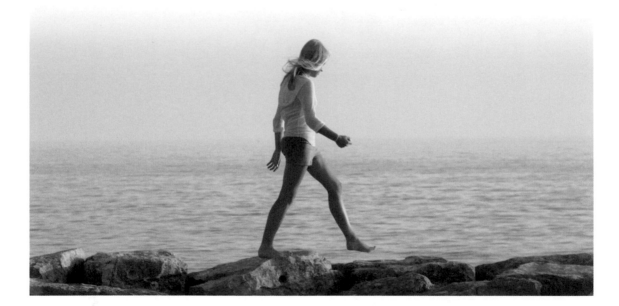

Exercising effortlessly

A pedometer measures the number of steps you take and can be a novice exerciser's best friend. Counting the steps you take each day is strangely compulsive, and equalling or bettering a previous score is a great incentive to doing more exercise.

Clip on your pedometer first thing in the morning and at the end of the day check how many steps you've taken. Was it an average day as far as activity is concerned? In that case, this is your 'base'. For most sedentary people it's around 2000–4000 steps per day. Experts tell us to aim for 10,000 steps a day – roughly 8 kilometres (5 miles), which is estimated to burn off approximately 500 calories. Once you know your base, then aim to increase that number by 1000 in the space of a week. If you carry on feeling well, then keep aiming for another 1000 each week until you reach the 10,000. If you suffer from discomfort or breathlessness, speak to your doctor.

Here are some ways to reach 10,000 steps:

• Pace while you're on the phone.

• Never use the remote control.

• Don't email colleagues – visit them at their desks.

• Walk round the playground while the children play.

• Pace while you're waiting for the bus or train.

• Use a loo on a different floor.

• Park in the bay furthest from the entrance to the building you're visiting.

• Run up and down the stairs during commercial breaks and while your computer is warming up.

• Don't use the nearest bus stop. Walk to the next one instead.

Clip your pedometer on the back of your waistband. It should be firmly attached because any place it jiggles around can cause it to overcount.

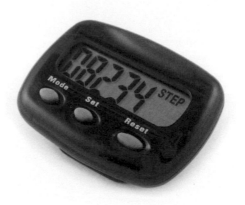

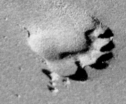

'If your aim is to lose body fat, begin with cardiovascular exercise. After developing a regular routine of two to three weeks, include some muscle conditioning exercise. With regular muscle conditioning exercise, you burn more calories all the time, even at rest, because your basal metabolic rate has been permanently raised with the increase of muscle.'

– LOUISE DAY, CHAMPNEYS' WELL-BEING DIRECTOR AND FITNESS EXPERT

Absolute beginners' programme
Start at whatever week (level) feels comfortable to you.

Week	Action	Number of times
Week: 1	Walk slowly for 5 minutes, briskly for 1 minute, slowly for 5 minutes	3 per week
Week: 2	Walk slowly for 5 minutes, briskly for 5 minutes, slowly for 5 minutes	5 per week
Week: 3	Walk slowly for 5 minutes, briskly for 10 minutes, slowly for 5 minutes	3 per week
Week: 4	Walk slowly for 5 minutes, briskly for 15 minutes, slowly for 5 minutes	5 per week

(Congratulations! You are now an official exerciser. At this level of activity, if you were not exercising before, you have increased your chances of living a longer life.)

Beginner's programme

Aim to walk for at least 30 minutes 4–5 times a week. After two weeks increase this to 30–45 minutes and work on improving your pace, increasing the number of steps you take per minute, the distance you cover and the number of hills you take on. All of these give you a better workout. Set yourself new goals to keep you interested.

(More congratulations. Taking an average thirty-minute walk most days of the week is reaching the level of exercise which has been shown to lower your cancer risk and your chance of heart and circulation disease, improve your chances of succumbing to depression and maintain strong bones.)

Calorie-blasting option
Try and fit in an hour of walking four times a week. The faster and further you walk the more calories you will be burning and the fitter you will become.

Move it up a gear

Hill walking

If your walking routine has become flat, pick it up with some hill walking. It will break the boredom and do away with the monotony of your workout. When you initially begin adding hills to your route, build slowly, adding more incline as you require increased intensity. Walking uphill will put a greater demand on the body because you're creating a bigger stretch in the ankle joint to walk up the incline. To ensure total success of this technique, focus on your posture and on having a strong centre to support your body.

Nordic walking

When you see walkers striding out, swinging two poles with each step, you're watching Nordic walking. Nordic walking was originally devised by cross-country skiers as a way to keep training during the summer when there was no snow. Now we know that the poles mean that Nordic walkers work harder than usual without feeling the strain. It is a brilliant way of pushing your walking workout to a new level.

- It burns up to 46% more calories than ordinary walking.

- It reduces tension in the neck and shoulders.

- It lessens the impact on the knees and joints.

To maximise the calorie burn and fitness benefits, it's best to learn how to do it properly from an instructor. In the UK visit www.nordicwalking.co.uk or call 020 8878 8108 to find your nearest instructor; elsewhere, just do a quick online search.

Nordic walking classes are available at Champneys Forest Mere and Champneys Tring.

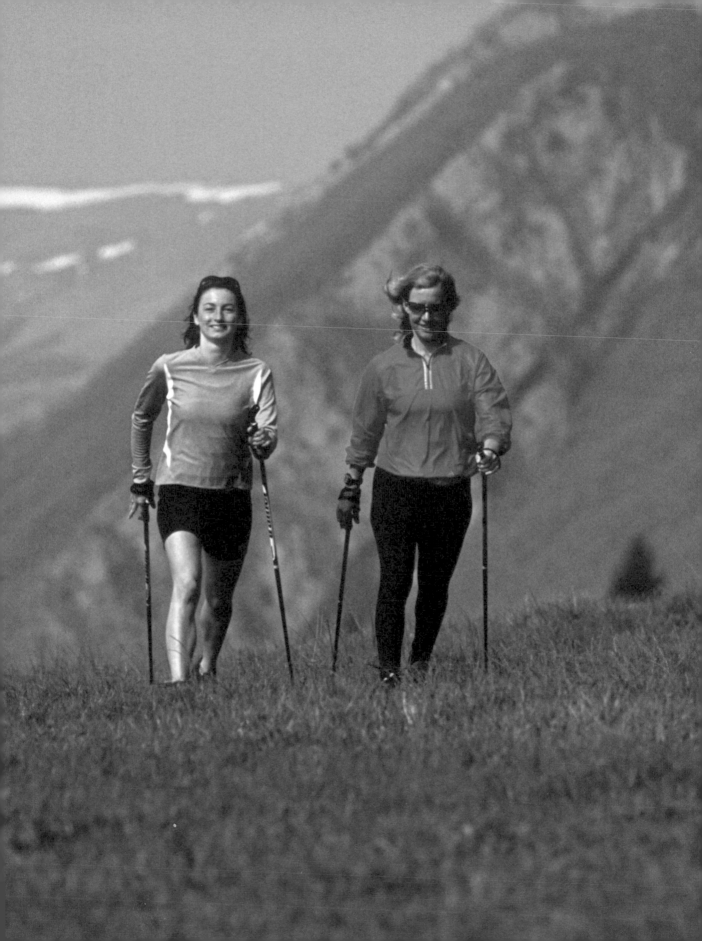

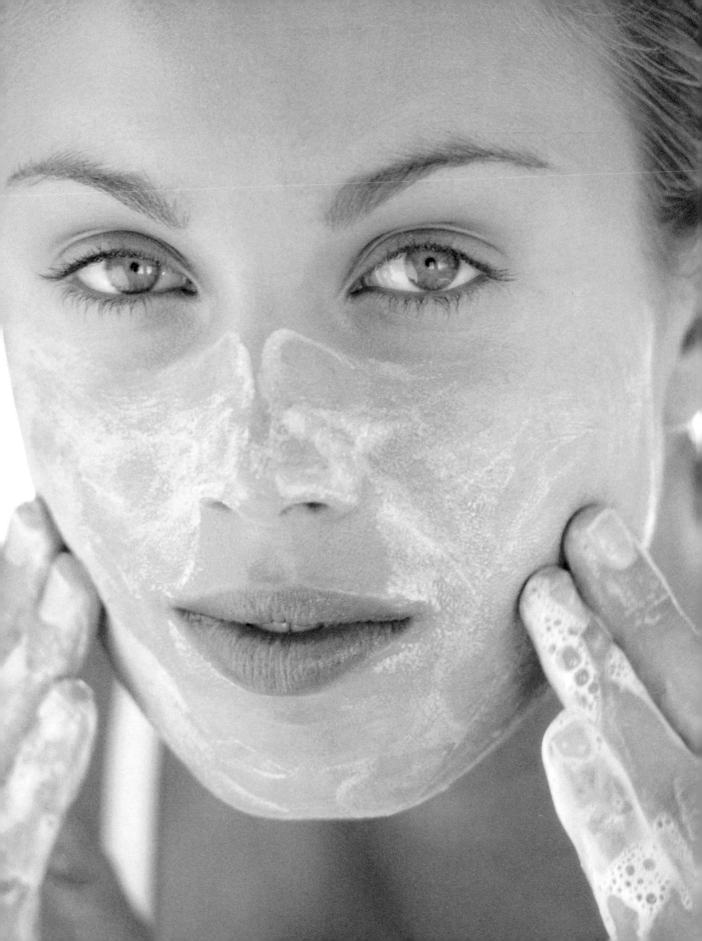

Love yourself

These treatments work well at any time but are especially suited to spring.

Polish and Purify Facial

This facial boosts the radiance of your skin. It revitalises your complexion and leaves your skin glowing. At Champneys, the facial uses micro-dermabrasion along with traditional steam and extraction to leave the skin refreshed and 'resurfaced'.

You'll need: cleanser, toner, a facial brush or flannel, a magnifying mirror, a micro-dermabrasion unit or product such as Champneys Micro-dermabrasion Facial Polish or Natural Micro-Derm Face Polish, a towel, cotton wool, eye and face masks, moisturiser, eye treatment.

Before you start: pour a pint of boiling water into a heat-proof bowl.

Cleanse and polish
Thoroughly cleanse your face of all make-up. Apply a foaming facial wash (such as Champneys Radiance Boosting Foamy Facial Wash) to your face and neck. Use a facial brush or Champneys Micro-Dermabrasion System to brush cleanse. Using a chamois or flannel and warm water, remove the foaming facial wash. Apply a gentle toner and then blot your face and neck with a man-size tissue.

Extract
Gently lower your face over the bowl of boiling water with a towel over your head. Do not let your face get too close to the water, remembering that steam can burn, too. (This is not recommended if you have visible broken capillaries.) Steam your face for a few minutes. Alternatively, if you're using a facial steamer unit, follow the manufacturer's guidelines. Blot with a tissue and wrap a tissue around each index finger. With any obvious blackheads, apply gentle pressure downwards on either side of the blocked pore. Do not do this over areas of broken capillaries or where skin is otherwise infected or broken.

Deep treat

After extraction, sweep a cotton pad soaked in toner over your face then blot with tissue. Next apply an eye mask such as Collagen Plus Anti-Wrinkle Eye Treatment, lip balm and a face mask. Smooth lotion on your hands and feet and lie down with your eyes closed for ten minutes.

Protect

Using a facial flannel, remove the masks and then sweep a cotton pad soaked in toner over your face again. Blot with a man-size tissue and apply moisturiser.

Citrus Body Glow

An invigorating full-body scrub and citrus body oil application that will stimulate dull, lifeless skin and leave your skin feeling smooth and conditioned. (It is a good treatment to do the day before applying self-tanning products.)

You'll need: citrus glow scrub in a small bowl, citrus-scented body wash, citrus-scented body oil, shower cap and a warm bathroom.

Before you start: Prepare the citrus products. Choose a citrus-scented scrub such as Champneys Citrus Sugar Scrub, or make your own by adding 10 drops of a citrus aromatherapy oil (e.g. bergamot, lemon, orange) to 10 ml of base oil (e.g. almond). Then add four large handfuls of caster sugar and mix everything to a paste. Use Champneys Citrus Glow Energising Shower Gel or customise your usual body wash (preferably a fragrance free one) by adding a few drops of aromatherapy oil, or by adding 10 drops to 20 ml of body oil.

Scrub

Tie your hair back and put on a shower cap. Standing in the bath or shower, using brisk, vigorous strokes, apply the scrub. Start at your back, then move to your arms, hips and buttocks, sweeping down to your ankles and the tops of your feet. Massage in the scrub over the entire body – except your face and neck.

Using the flat of the palm, rub the scrub over your legs and feet one more time. Lift your right arm above your head and massage with the left hand, then lift your left arm above your head and massage with the right hand.

Starting from the navel, one hand following the other, make a big, circular, clockwise motion. Place both hands over the base of your breastbone and sweep them down to your ribs, then down to below the navel in a diamond shape. Again, repeat this six times.

Place both hands over the base of your breastbone again then, in a cross-heart movement, alternate your hands under the bust, finishing at the opposite shoulder. Repeat six times.

Cross your arms over your chest and press down hard on the opposite shoulder. Breathe in the scent of the citrus to 'ground' you. Then shower off the scrub with a citrus-scented body wash using circular movements.

Massage

Pat yourself dry lightly and massage in a citrus-scented body oil starting with your back (as much as you can, or find a helper), buttocks and legs; then move to the arms, stomach and bust. Place a towel on your bed and lie down to let the oil soak in. Relax and inhale the scent – place another towel or sheet over your body if it's cool. You should feel relaxed but invigorated after this treatment.

> '*Why do we pay for psychotherapy, when massage costs half as much.*'
> - JASON LOVE, AMERICAN HUMORIST

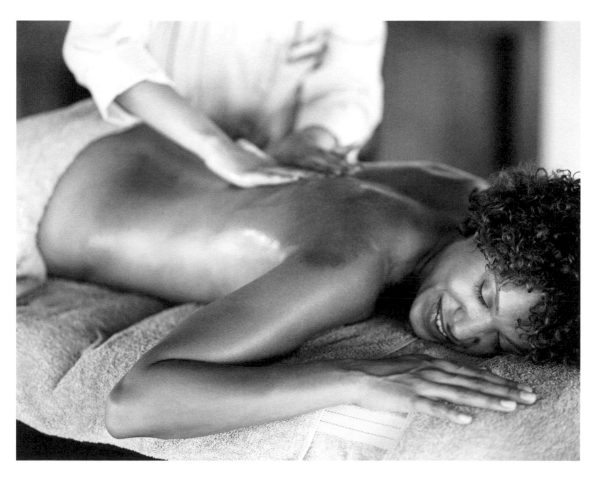

The instant confidence booster

A tan is great for confidence. You look longer, leaner, more toned – and all without much effort. Faking it is so much safer than baking in the sun. These days self tans are sophisticated, easy to use, quick drying and incredibly effective. They come in mousses, creams, gels, sprays and lotions. You can apply them yourself – home tans tend to last up to five days – or you can go the professional route and visit a specialist salon. Salon tans tend to last longer, perhaps for a week to a fortnight. The best salon treatments include St. Tropez, Elemis, La Prairie, Daphine, Guinot and Clarins. Many self tans take a few days to look natural so if you're preparing for a special day, book your treatment a few days in advance.

You can fake a tan at home. Follow Champneys' golden rules:

- Exfoliate. Use a body scrub and loofah to slough off dead skin. Concentrate on areas where hard skin is rougher, such as knees, elbows and feet.

- Moisturise. Leave a body lotion on for fifteen minutes before you apply self tan so it doesn't interfere with the active ingredient in the tanning product. Oil cuticles on hands and feet. Blot this off with a damp flannel before you apply the tanning product, especially on bony areas, to prevent uneven streaks.

- Layer. Apply the self tan as you would a moisturiser. Be careful to make a smooth application over the backs of knees and hands and anywhere where the tan may concentrate. Apply the main bulk of product to the larger surface areas, such as the middle of your thigh and then lightly go over areas like the knees to prevent this area going too dark. The colour usually appears about three or four hours later. If you have streaks, try exfoliating – or you can buy special products that help remove them.

- Avoid swimming or showering for twelve hours.

- Moisturise your body every day to prolong your tan.

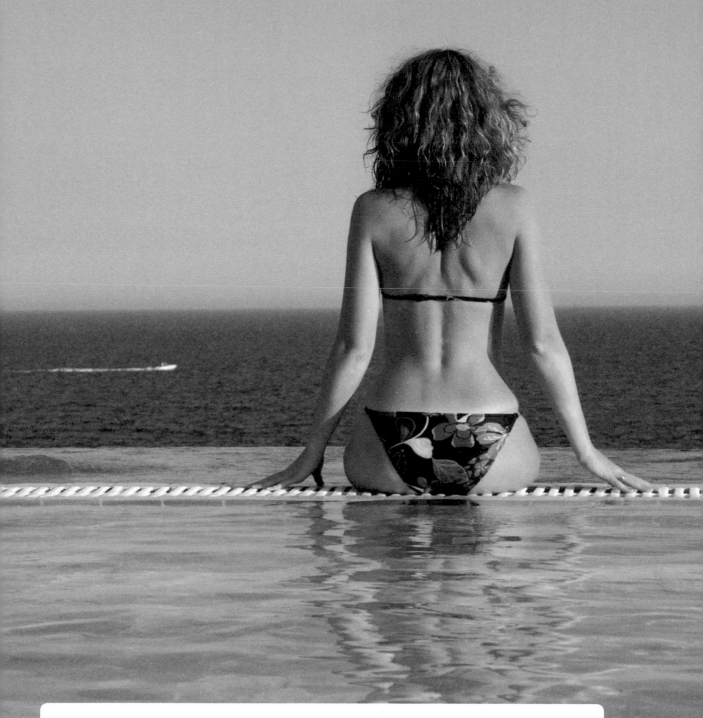

Wash your hands immediately after applying self tan to prevent orange palms developing. If your hands are discoloured, rub them with lemon juice and then wash your hair. Doing both will help to remove the stains. Champneys Manicure Miracle Softening Scrub will also help with removal of any stains.

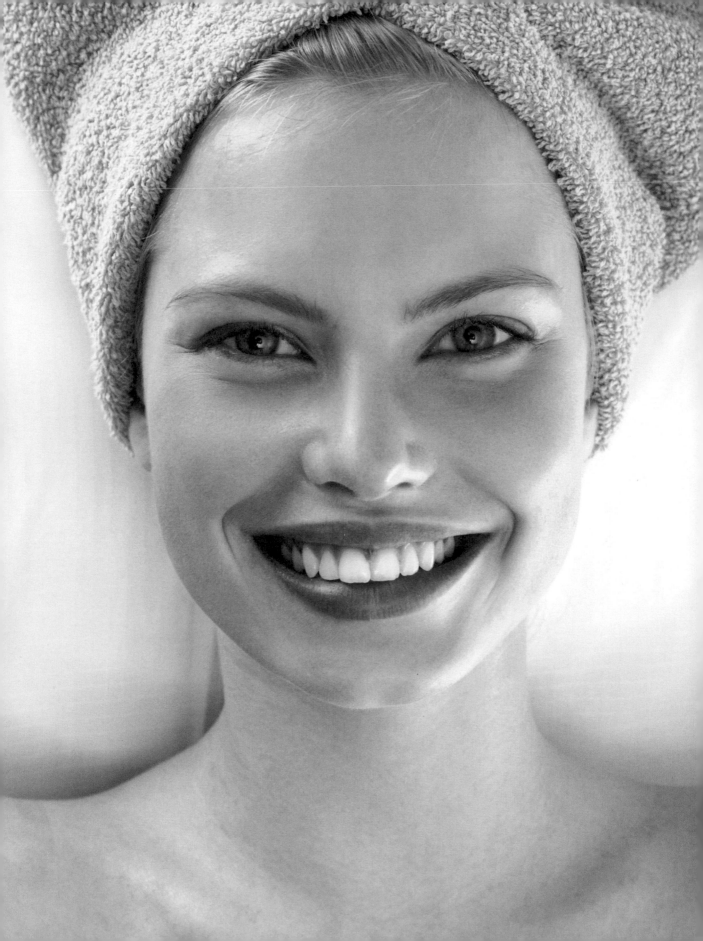

Bright Eyes

This decongesting eye treatment will revitalise tired, puffy eyes and plump out any fine lines using a collagen eye mask – as well as leaving you feeling totally relaxed.

You'll need: a couple of pillows for under your knees, a blanket, cotton wool, a flannel or facial cloth and man-sized tissues.

Before you start: collect all you need for the treatment and do a 'dry run' with the instructions to get the hang of the intricate movements. This treatment is much more relaxing if you can lie down with pillows under your knees while doing it. Cleanse your skin of all make-up and tie your hair back.

Apply facial oil to your face
Using the middle and ring fingers of each hand, and starting between the brows at the place sometimes called the 'third eye', make slow, firm circular motions out to the temples, then under your eyes coming up to the 'third eye' and finishing at the temples again. Circle, pressing gently on the temples, six times. Repeat the entire movement three times.

Finger press release
Using your index finger, glide to the outer corner of the eye. Press and release to get to the inner corner, glide up the side of your nose and circle at the temples. Repeat three times.

Thumb press release
From your temples, move your thumbs to the inside corner of your eyes. Using the thumbs, press and release. Take one thumb off at a time and place at the 'third eye'. Press and release and work out towards the temples. Repeat three times.

Circle with fingertips at the temples three times.

Hook and wave
Place both of your index fingers at your 'third eye' and pull them along the brow line, then use first and second, then all three fingers in a wave movement across the brow line. Repeat three times.

57

Circle with fingertips at the temples three times. Then, with your ring finger supported by the middle finger, glide to the outer corner of the eye and make small circles to the inner corner, glide up the side of the nose, circle at the 'third eye', drain over eyebrows and repeat the sequence three times.

With your ring finger supported by the middle finger, circle at the temples, starting with firm pressure and getting lighter and lighter until your fingers gently lift off your forehead at the temples.

Relax

Apply an eye mask, and two pads of cotton wool soaked in cool water, to your eyes.
Relax for ten minutes, then remove the pads and eye mask.

Fold a tissue into three and place it across both eyes, place your hands – with three fingers facing inwards – on top; press and release.

Moisturise

Apply moisturiser to your face and neck, circle at the temples using firm pressure, again getting lighter and lighter until you lift your fingers off at the temples. Relax some more.

Express French manicure

You will need: cuticle stick, emery board or nail file, buffer, nail clippers.
Before you start: Fill a bowl with warm water.

Clip your nails into a neat shape and file them, but in one direction only – do not saw at them. Put your fingers into the bowl of warm water and soak your nails for a minute, then remove your hands and dry them thoroughly.

Apply a drop of oil to each cuticle and massage it in. Gently ease back the cuticles of each nail with an orange stick using small circular movements.

Apply a good hand and nail cream, such as Champneys Age Excellence Ultimate Hand Treatment, to the hands and forearms. Massage each hand and forearm three times. Clean under the nails with the other end of the orange stick. Then apply your nail varnish over one layer of base coat.

How to do a natural French polish.

Apply a base coat. Apply one coat of pale French polish, either pink or natural, then carefully apply the white starting at the far side, doing one continuous line across. You can use guide strips which stick onto the nail to help create a perfect line. These must only be put onto dry polish and it is also advisable to wait until the white is dry before you remove the strip. Finish with a clear top coat.

When your nails are totally dry, apply a product such as Champneys Nail and Cuticle Wonder Oil (or a similar nourishing oil), one drop to each cuticle. Massage it in well.

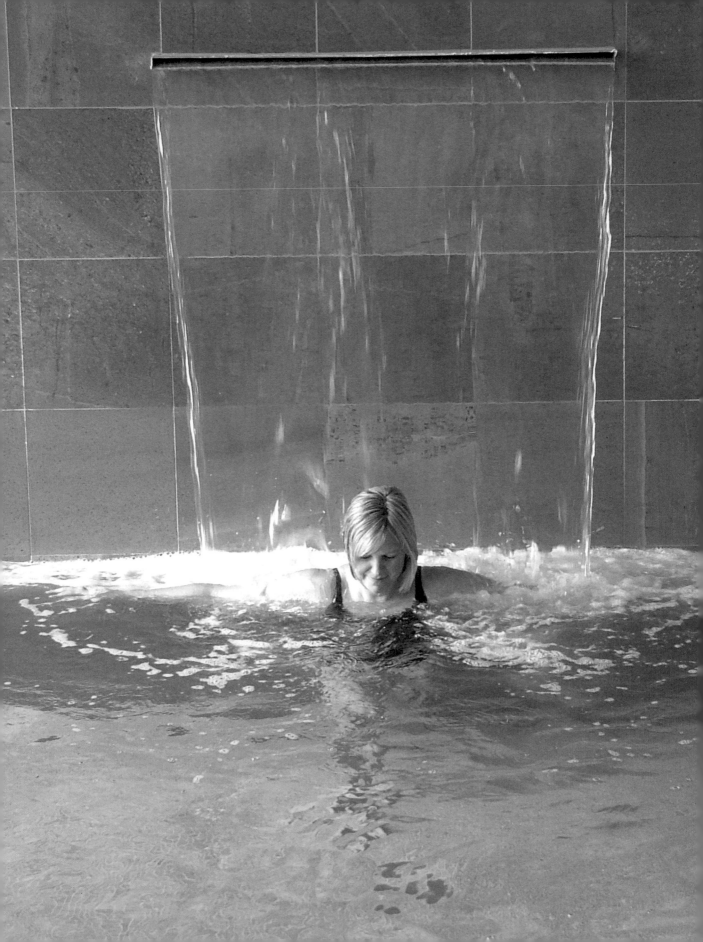

Well-being

Detox your life

Spring is a great time to re-evaluate how you spend your time, and who you spend it with. (Hint: it's not just our bodies that could do with detoxing.)

Some people are energy black holes. They suck the happiness and cheer out of your day. They have their own agenda and you can have no idea what that is, let alone do anything about it. All you can do, when you meet a stranger determined to rain on your parade, is to imagine yourself in an impervious bubble of white light and keep smiling through. They will pass from your life soon. But what do you do when the black hole is one of your inner circle? What do you do when you share a life, a home, a bed with an energy drainer?

Don't waste a minute dwelling on how much better life would be if your partner would only be kinder or your mum would cheer up a bit, if your teenagers were more polite or your boss less of an idiot. You can't do anything to change their behaviour. You can only alter how you interact with them.

Try this. Take a piece of paper and list the people with whom you have most contact. Then divide the list into three categories:

• **The Energisers.** They make you feel great. They give great advice. They bring joy.

• **The Neutral.** They are just there.

• **The Drainers.** Sometimes they are nice people but just a little bit wearing. They always seem to have a problem. They always seem to be low. It can be worse – they could be users, people who don't deliver, let you down, bring you down. They also include gossips, bitches (of both sexes), sarcastic types whose conversation, although funny, leaves you feeling a bit tacky afterwards.

This exercise can be really illuminating. You can see at a glance where your energy may be expended unwisely – basically, propping up those who aren't giving enough back. On the other hand, you can see at a moment if there are enough Energisers in your life, and if not, why not? Make it your practice to spot the Energisers when you walk into a room. Gravitate towards them, nurture your friendships with them.

If, by chance, the Drainers in your life are those people you spend the most time with, be aware of how much their mood impacts on you. Refuse to be drawn into their world. Move away when it feels like too much. By withdrawing when they become negative, you give them the chance to raise their game.

Look through your diary for the last few months. How much of your time was spent on tasks that drained you of energy or fitted in with other people's agendas? When you are scheduling over the next few months, be conscious of whether the activity you're considering is really worth the effort in terms of enjoyment or payback to you. Just thinking a little more about what you agree to can make a radical difference to how much time you have for the activities that replenish you.

Finally, spring clean. Throw out everything you don't need or use any more. This creates space in your life (literally) and in your mind. You will find it easier to keep to new habits when your life is clear of clutter.

'No matter how much I have to do, as soon as I walk into one of our resorts, I calm right down. I begin to walk more slowly – and that immediately has a calming effect. Try walking slowly but purposefully the next time you're stressed out. You might find it works for you, too.'

– JO PARKER, CHAMPNEYS' SPA DIRECTOR AND BEAUTY EXPERT

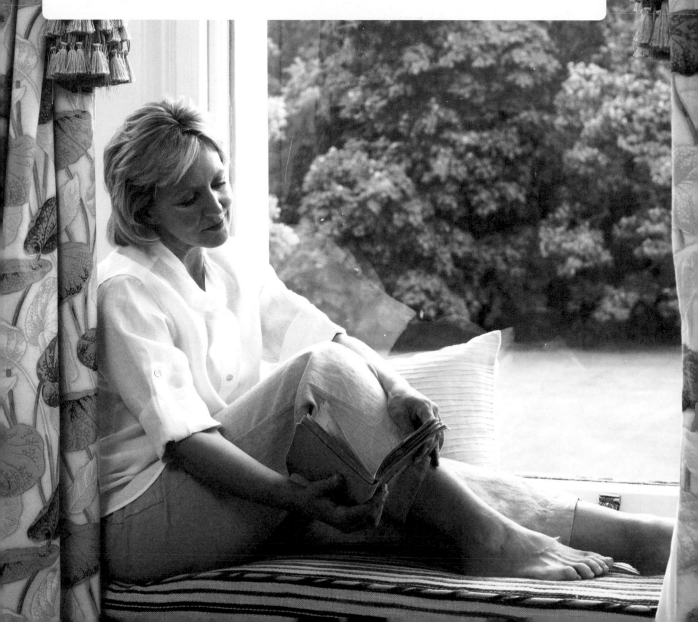

Create your own sacred space

Take time to create your own 'sanctuary'. A room, a corner, or simply a comfortable chair where you can retreat to relax and take stock. When creating your sanctuary think in terms of stimulating your senses: choose a lovely view or place objects you love to gaze on nearby, have favourite music to hand and a luxurious throw to snuggle into, burn favourite oils or candles while you relax…

Just a few minutes in your sanctuary each day will chill you out – and the effects are cumulative. The more time you spend there, the more quickly you'll respond to its power to calm you right down.

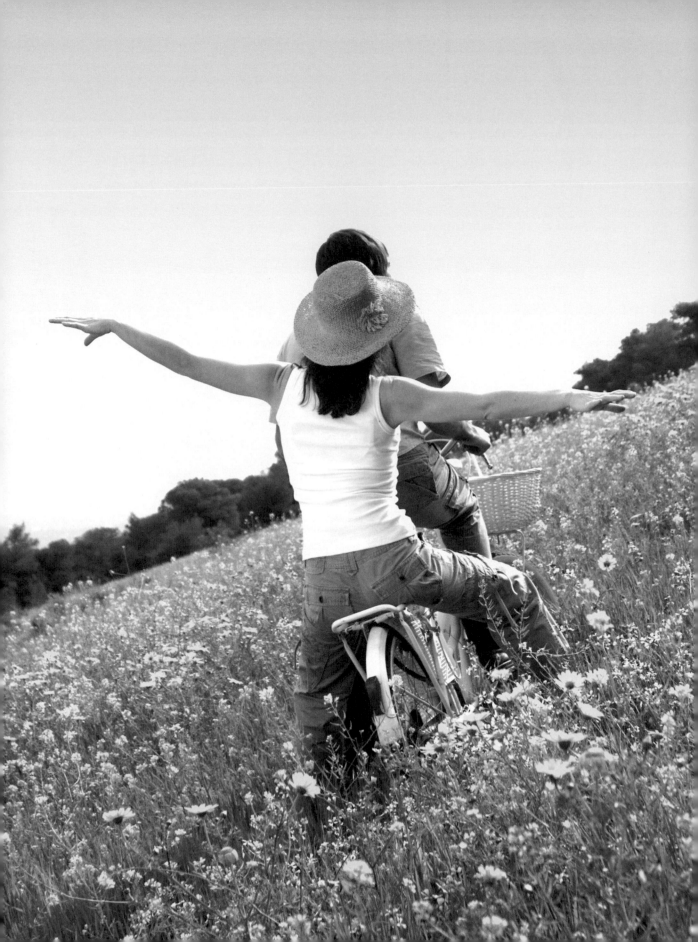

Escape – Be rejuvenated

Are you feeling frazzled, tired, sluggish or bloated after winter? Then ease into a new way of living with the Champneys' rejuvenation programme. At heart it's a detox – but a gentle one. Do not think of it as an extreme regime, as it's more of a non-tox than a detox. The aim is to give your body a holiday from the stresses of twenty-first century living by eating plenty of the food that is easiest for it to digest while undergoing restorative treatments.

The point is not to lose weight (although that is a bonus if you have a few pounds to lose after winter), but to give your body a break so that you'll experience a boost in vitality, improve circulation, and look radiant and relaxed.

The whole concept of detoxing has its critics – our bodies are perfectly capable of dealing with any 'toxins', they argue. To an extent that's true, but with one caveat: we have never been exposed to so many toxins before. One definition of toxin is any chemical substance that can adversely affect the health if a person is exposed to it too much, and they include pollutants, additives, smoke, caffeine and alcohol. On top of that, we all sleep less than previous generations did, and sleep is essential for regeneration.

Champneys' three-day rejuvenation programme combats the effects of our normal life…

What's lymph got to do with it?

Lymph does for your body what dustbin men do for your home – it takes away the rubbish. Think of your lymphatic system as being similar to your circulatory system – a vast, intricate network of tiny vessels that dispose of bacteria, dead cells, toxins and anything else that you need to get rid of. The lymph system transports this debris to the lymph nodes which are concentrated in the groin, armpits, knees and under the jaw. There it is attacked and disposed of by the white blood cells. When people talk of 'boosting your immune system', they are in part talking about supporting your lymph system. Infection finds it hard to take hold when the lymph system is working well. Other benefits are a clear skin and even less of a propensity to cellulite. Any puffiness, swollen ankles or eyes or frequent colds are a sign that lymph isn't working well.

Strategies that will help your lymph system

• One of the great advantages of detoxing is that your lymph system really benefits from the changes you make. Eating easily digested food, free of additives and pesticides, gives lymph less to do, and exercising helps it flow freely.

• Skin brushing boosts lymph circulation. Using a natural bristle brush or exfoliating mitts, sweep your dry skin prior to taking a shower or bath. Start at your toes, move to the top of your feet, up legs and to your buttocks, then do your fingers, hands and arms.

Always work towards your heart until every part of you has been brushed (except your face). This boosts circulation and makes your skin glow. It is also strangely compulsive, and soon you will feel that you are not bathing properly without skin brushing first.

• If you are really serious about detoxing, try this famous liver tonic which combines citrus with healthy oils: squeeze the juice of two oranges and one lemon into a glass and add a crushed clove of garlic, some finely chopped ginger and one tablespoon of extra virgin olive oil. Stir vigorously and drink first thing in the morning.

• Rosemary aromatherapy essential oil is invigorating to the lymph. Add a few drops to a warm bath and get in, then allow it to cool right down. Your circulation, including that of lymph, is aided by the change in temperature.

• Massage. This also boosts the circulation. Self-massage with rosemary oil diluted in a carrier oil is great for this, or book yourself in for a special kind of massage known as manual lymphatic drainage (MLD). Gentle press and release movements move the lymph along.

(The 'Bright Eyes' treatment on page 57 uses MLD movements to decongest the eye area.)

Are you at risk of toxic overload?

How much would you benefit from detoxing? Our quiz opposite will give you some indication. Score one point for each 'a', two for each 'b' and three for every 'c' to discover how 'toxed' you are right now…

1. Do you smoke?

a) Never ☐

b) I'm a social smoker ☐

c) Most days ☐

2. Do you drink alcohol?

a) Never ☐

b) On average, one glass a day ☐

c) More than one glass a day on average ☐

3. Do you eat ready meals and takeaways?

a) Two times a month or less ☐

b) Three or four times a month ☐

c) Twice or more a week on average ☐

4. How much water do you drink?

a) Two litres a day ☐

b) Several glasses ☐

c) I know it's not enough ☐

5. Do you live or work where there is a lot of traffic?

a) No ☐

b) I live or work near traffic but not both ☐

c) I live and work near traffic ☐

6. How often do you feel jittery, stressed and on edge?

a) Hardly ever – can't remember the last time ☐

b) About once a month ☐

c) Once or more a week ☐

7. Do you exercise in a 'fresh air' environment?

a) Several times a week ☐

b) Several times a month ☐

c) Less than that ☐

8. Are you prone to colds and flu?

a) Hardly ever ☐

b) Twice a year or so ☐

c) More than that ☐

8–12: Your lifestyle is healthy already and you may not feel the need for the rejuvenation programme. But if you are tired, you might find that the programme gives you a lift.

13–18: Your health and well-being would benefit from the programme but it would be worthwhile taking the time to prepare for it particularly well and make it sabotage-free. That's because although you try hard to live healthily, life has a habit of getting in the way.

19–24: The rejuvenation programme might be difficult for you to follow as it will probably require several key changes. The good news is that you will benefit the most from giving your body a break.

This will work best if you can clear three days in your diary to take it easy and concentrate on resting when you feel like it. You may be making big changes in your diet and that can be tiring.

If you drink a lot of coffee or other caffeinated drinks, then begin to cut down prior to the programme: this will minimise the risk of withdrawal headaches when you give up during the programme. Follow the eating tips on page 20–22 as much as possible.

An even quicker test?
Invest in Champneys Detox Patches. These are worn on the soles of your feet and draw toxins out overnight. The darker they are, the more you might benefit from supplementing their action with the rejuvenation programme.

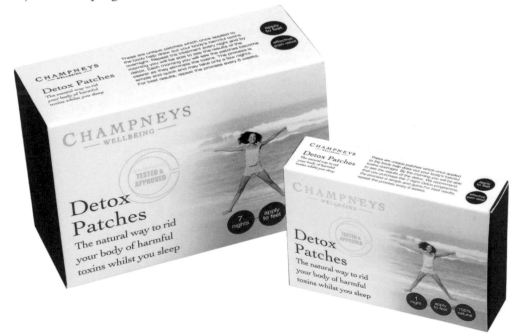

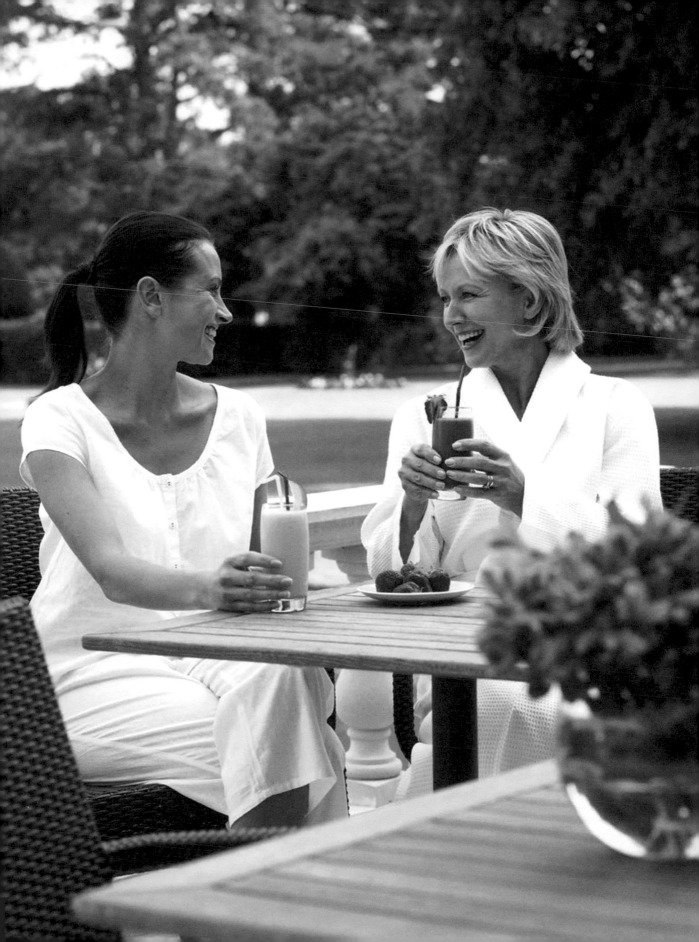

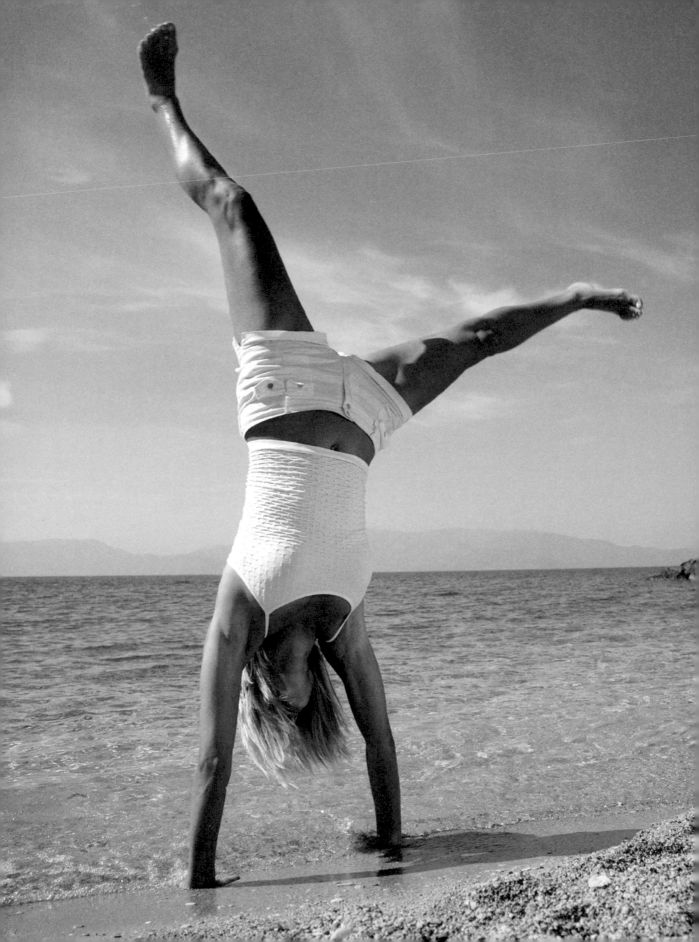

The Champneys' three-day rejuvenation programme

What not to eat – and what you can eat: the inner cleanse

Our bodies have efficient systems for dealing with waste products. The key players are the organs of elimination (bowels, skin, kidneys, lungs) and liver. The purpose of the inner cleanse is to support them.

In the early days of Champneys, under the watchful eye of the founder, renowned naturopath Stanley Lief, residents reported an increase in vitality after a regime of very strict limitation of their food intake. Fasting is still seen as the classic 'detox' diet but now we recognise that fasting is not for everyone and that some people feel worse rather than better after fasting. Champneys offer a gentler regime – a low tox rather than a detox, a diet packed with vital nutrients necessary to support the body's ability to heal itself.

The body breaks down, processes and transforms substances that it ingests. Well over half of this activity involves substances which could be harmful. The liver does this through a process called 'conjugation'. The principle is to avoid food and drink that increase the liver's workload.

How to eat

- Meals should be regular – three a day, and a mid-morning and mid-afternoon snack.
- Eat moderate helpings of good lean protein with main meals: fish, eggs, chicken, tofu. The size of your palm is a good guide to your protein portion size.
- Dandelion coffee, ginger (in ginger tea, or added to juice or food) and nettle tea are all good for cleansing/supporting the liver.

Here's an example of how it might work:

Breakfast

To a small bowl of porridge made with water, add blueberries (frozen are fine), walnuts and some plain organic soya yoghurt, or have a poached egg and cooked tomatoes on a slice of rye bread, with a small glass of pomegranate or purple grape juice.

Lunch

Make a large rainbow salad of vegetables (include broccoli, watercress, avocado and spinach leaves to support organs of elimination). Add protein: some fish (tinned sardines or salmon are fine), an egg or some organic tofu. Dress with some olive oil and lemon juice. Finish by having some melon and an apple.

Dinner

Grilled chicken or fish, lots of steamed vegetables (a rainbow of colours to maximise nutrient content) and a helping of sweet potato, with mashed celeriac or Puy lentils. End with a few Brazil nuts.

Snacks

Nibble fruit and a few nuts or seeds.

Three pills worth popping

Good quality supplements will help support your detox.

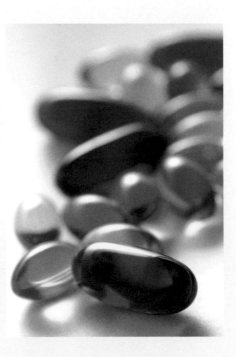

- A good basic multivitamin/mineral to ensure that you have all the vitamins and minerals to aid the detoxification processes.

- A probiotic – 'good' bacteria to support intestinal and liver health. Look for one which also contains FOS (fructo-oligosaccharides) which beneficial bacteria use as substrate (food) and which encourage their growth.

- Look for a good detox supplement containing glutathione/MSM which supports the liver's detoxification pathways.

No	Yes
• No alcohol. • No processed food – that means no foods that have been modified by man. So no hydrogenated fats in margarines, biscuits and cakes, artificial sweeteners, additives and preservatives. No fried food, either. • No sugar. • No red meat. • No caffeinated drinks. • No wheat or dairy foods (which are common causes of food sensitivity and more difficult to digest). • Very little salt.	• Include foods (organic if possible) that nourish your body. • Drink plenty of water and herbal teas – at least 2 litres a day. • Eat plenty of vegetables (except white potatoes). These are especially good for detox: artichokes, beetroot, bean and seed sprouts, carrots, pumpkin, red cabbage, spinach, sweet potato, tomato, watercress. Cruciferous vegetables – broccoli, cauliflower, kale, cabbage, Brussels sprouts – are particularly important in supporting the key conjugation pathways in the liver. • Eat fruit. Especially good for detoxing: apples, fresh apricots, berries, cantaloupe melon, citrus, kiwi, papaya, peaches, mango and dark grapes. • Grains – a half tennis-ball sized helping of brown rice, corn, millet, oats or quinoa. • Pulses. • Nuts and seeds (great for snacks with some fruit). • Oils – use extra virgin olive oil or flaxseed oil.

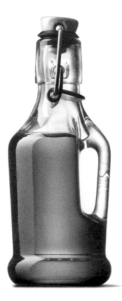

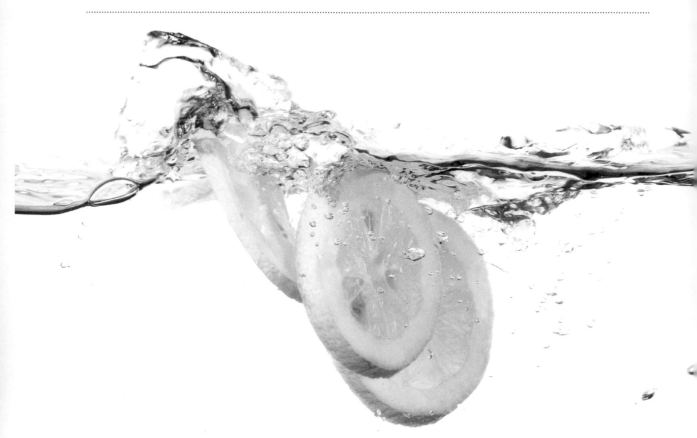

Why lemon water?

Each morning, start the day with half a lemon squeezed into a glass of hot water. During the night, our livers are busy processing all that we have ingested the day before. Lemon promotes liver function and is an ancient method of aiding the liver in its essential work.

Here are some routines to help, too:

Day 1
First thing: Lemon water.
Before you shower or bathe: Skin brushing.
During the day: A brisk walk to aid circulation
Treatment: Polish and Purify.
Bed: Try to be in bed by 10 p.m. Read or listen to restful music if you can't sleep.

Day 2
First thing: Lemon water.
Before you shower or bathe: Skin brushing.
During the day: A brisk walk to aid circulation.

Treatment: Citrus Body Glow.

Bed: Aim to be in bed by 9.30 p.m. Adopt the yoga pose of the child beforehand to help relax you (see the illustration on page 255). Kneel on the floor and bend forward so that your chest rests on your knees but your bottom stays as close as possible to your heels (you may want to put a folded towel under your forehead). Your arms should point backwards with the back of your hands resting on the floor, palm upwards. Feel the pull along your spine. Let your muscles 'drop' downwards. Breathe normally, but on the out breath, concentrate on releasing tension. Maintain this position for several minutes or as long as is comfortable.

Day 3

First thing: Lemon water.

Before you shower or bathe: Skin brushing.

During the day: A brisk walk to aid circulation.

Treatment: Bright Eyes.

Before bed: Adopt the child's pose again and aim to be in bed by 10 p.m.

Summer

Five ways to celebrate summer

- Sink into a lavender bath. Bathing in lavender is deeply relaxing. It calms your busy mind and soothes you off to sleep. Make your own lavender infusion by soaking half a cup of lavender blossoms in a cup of boiling water and then filtering it into your bath water, or treat yourself to Champneys Perfect Sleep Bath Milk and Perfect Sleep Pillow Mist.

- Relax with flowers. Turn flower arranging into a relaxing ritual. Instead of flinging flowers randomly into a vase, take time to select blooms and visualise the finished effect, spend time touching, smelling and enjoying the flowers. Experiment with single stems rather than a whole bunch. See it as a creative meditation.

- Play more. Splash with the kids in the paddling pool, challenge your partner to a water fight, take on friends at tennis at the weekend. We are hardwired to get outside and have fun in summer – just think what a relief and release the summer months must have been for our ancestors. It's good for our mood and it's good for our relationships. (A connection has been made between the end of playfulness in couples' relationships and the onset of marital discord.)

- Celebrate Midsummer Day. Throw a pagan party. Rejoice in all things alternative and chip in for an astrologer or tarot reader to entertain you. Even better, book a reflexologist or massage therapist.

- Walk tall. How is your posture? If you slouch, think about some Alexander Technique classes to help your posture. You'll feel better and look far more elegant on the beach when you're 'posture perfect'.

It's your time to shine

June is a great month to seek out a free cosmetics makeover at your local beauty counter. Summer make-up should be lighter and simpler (and remember, wearing the same make-up all year can be ageing). You might learn some fabulous new tricks.

July is a great month to invite your girlfriends over for a spa party. Choose a theme – Moroccan harem, summer beach, cosmopolitan chic. Use this book as inspiration; the treatments are even more relaxing when you aren't the one doing the treating.

August is a great month to have an outdoor mud bath. One warm day, slather yourself in a mud or a clay body mask and lie on the grass until it dries. Sponge it off or, even better, if you have children get them to hose you down. Great for your circulation.

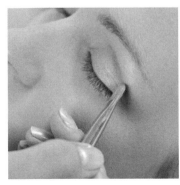 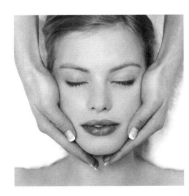 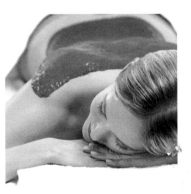

June... July... August... Summer

Relax... summer is here. Time to kick back, cut loose, live free.

Lose yourself... on balmy nights and sunny days. Stay up late to count the stars, even later to greet the dawn.

Reconnect... with friends and your younger, more carefree self; remember the thrill of being seventeen on a hot summer night.

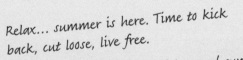

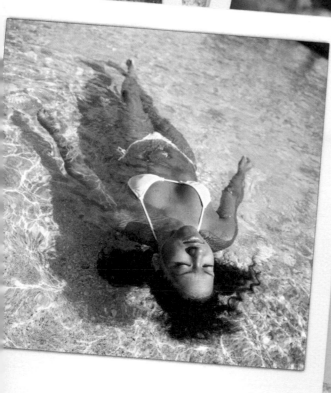

Immerse… in aquamarine water, lavender baths, sunsets on the beach, a really good book in the back garden and a cool glass of wine.

Remember… what really matters to you in life.

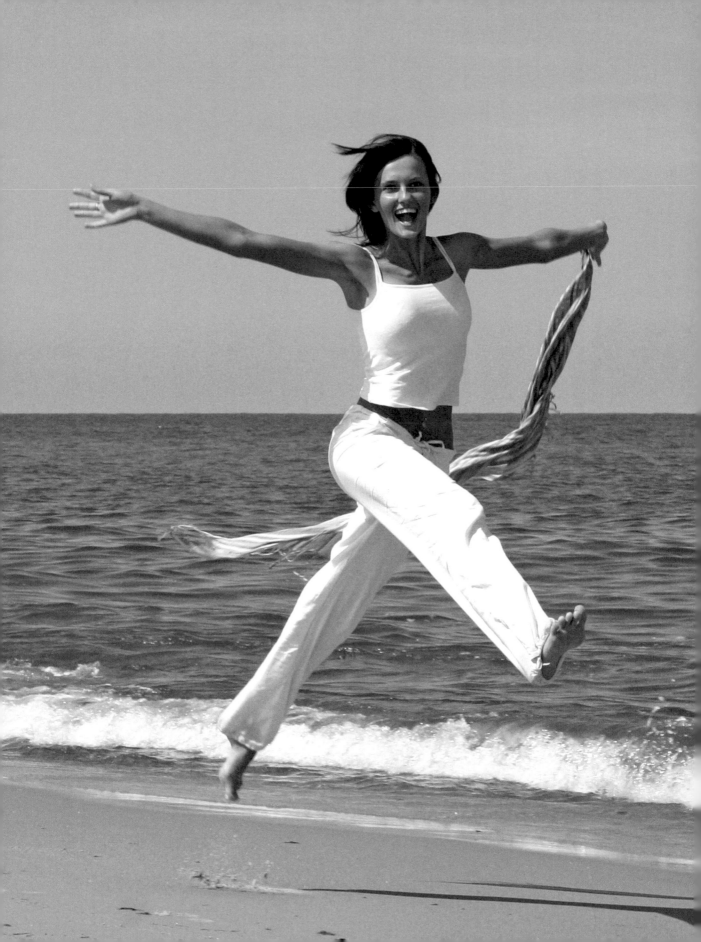

Eat

Time to get strong, time to get beautiful

Strong… toned… supple. Whatever you would most love for your body becomes not just possible, but probable, in summer. Now is the time to nurture, nourish and revel in the skin you were born in. Time to thank your amazing body for all it does for you with the movement, nutrition and pampering treatments that will have it purring like a well-oiled engine.

And besides rewarding your body, there are benefits for your self-esteem too. Summer means body consciousness. We wear less, we're on show more. We wouldn't be human if we didn't want to look good. As the temperature rises, and we emerge from beneath our winter layers, it's the time of the year when we start contemplating our navel – literally.

Let's build on the themes first explored in spring but move up a gear and start looking for the sort of results in terms of fitness and diet that will have you looking and feeling terrific through this summer – and, if you stick with them, for the rest of your life.

Losing weight – if you need to, now is the time

Summer is the ideal time for anyone to lose weight. The outdoors calls us to get outside and move, and the foods we're drawn to are just the ones that help us lose a few pounds without feeling for a minute that we're missing out.

Calorie counting is not the focus of weight management at Champneys. Of course, it's a fact that if you eat more calories than you use, you will put on weight, but we also know that women can be obsessed with calories and still put on weight.

Looking at the science in more depth helps us find the answers. The balance of food groups, in particular managing the amount and type of carbohydrate-rich foods is a key issue for most overweight people. That's because carb-rich foods have an impact on the body's ability to burn fat, which is vital for weight management. Inhibit fat burning, and fat stores accumulate. And that's exactly what happens in someone who eats more carbohydrate-rich foods than their body needs.

Carbohydrates are easily converted to energy. But carbohydrate in excess of our energy needs is converted to fat by insulin and stored in the fat cells, so the fat stores grow.

We differ in how we respond to carbohydrate depending on genetics, activity levels and the amount of fat we already have. In one UK study, a group of women were studied for the ease with which their bodies turned carbohydrates into fat. Lean women didn't make this conversion particularly easily. When both groups ate more carbohydrate than was needed to meet their energy requirements, the overweight women turned carbohydrate into fat three times as easily. So what can be done about it…

Our DNA was designed for a hunter-gatherer diet, mainly protein and plant foods, nuts and seeds. The sources included fruit and vegetables rather than cereals and grains. Wheat, rice and other grains are relatively recent additions to our diet in evolutionary terms. Also, until very recently in history, grains were ground between a couple of stones rather than over-processed and refined.

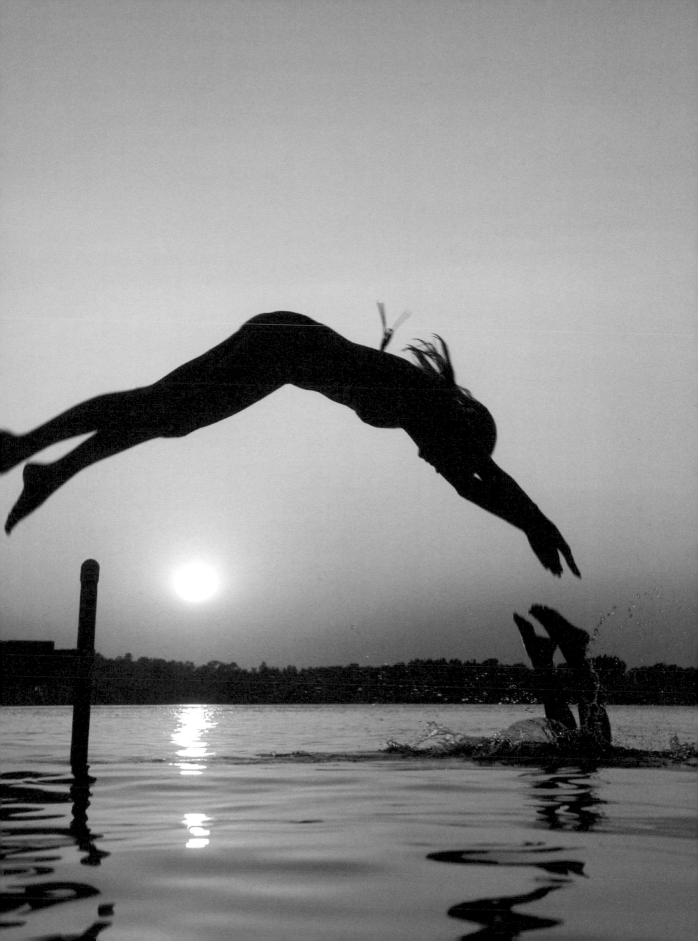

Losing weight – why it's worth it...

Being overweight wrecks your health. Even if on the outside you look healthy, fatty deposits will already be distributed around your organs and your blood pressure may be high. If you have a lot of weight to lose it can be disheartening to even get started, but even tiny losses in weight can result in better health and lengthen your life. Lose just 5–10% of your body weight and you'll reduce your risk of a whole host of diseases, from diabetes to heart disease, plus minor aches and pains will just disappear. Losing just half a kilo (about a pound) a week could result in a loss of 26 kilos over a whole year – and that's about 4 stones...

Research shows that the incidence of health problems due to increased weight rises almost in line with the amount of weight you put on rather than how long you have been at a particular weight. In other words, no matter how long you've been overweight, the risks diminish as soon as you start losing weight.

The science bit

Carbohydrates have been classified by scientists into the Glycaemic Index (GI). You will almost certainly have heard of this but may not know the details, or how it can help. The GI is a measure of how quickly foods are absorbed into the blood stream and so trigger insulin, and can be used to compare different foods. The faster something is absorbed, the higher its GI. Higher GI foods don't keep blood-sugar levels stable and a quick energy boost is followed by a slump, leaving you craving more. Those with a low GI rating keep you fuller for longer and keep cravings at bay. Moderate GI foods can be enjoyed in controlled amounts as part of a balanced meal.

Four kinds of food are **carbohydrate-rich**:

1. **Starchy vegetables**, mostly roots. White potatoes (baked potatoes in particular) are often perceived as an ideal 'diet' food, but this is not the case. They have a higher GI.

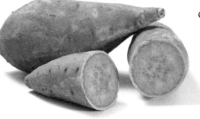

2. **Pulses** – beans, peas, lentils. These are a good choice of carb-rich food, and most have a moderate GI.

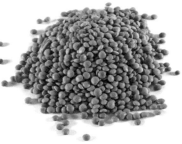

3. **Grains.** These can have a high GI, so avoid things like over-processed breakfast cereals.

4. **Fruit** is carb-rich and, unlike other food types, is pure carbohydrate. The sugars it contains give it its sweet taste. The best choices are lower-sugar fruits (which have less of an impact on blood sugar) including berries, apples, pears, grapefruit and plums. Dried fruit, fruit juice and shop-bought smoothies are all blood-sugar boosters, so are best left off the menu for now.

The GI doesn't take into account portion size. A more useful measure, which combines the GI of a food and a relevant portion size, is the Glycaemic Load or GL. Working with the GL rather than GI means you eat sufficient good-quality carbohydrate to keep your mood steady and cravings at bay – but that carbohydrate is unlikely to contribute to your fat stores.

At Champneys we recommend understanding and using the concept of Glycaemic Load to those people who want to lose weight. The best friend for them is the Champneys' light diet plate: GI + Champneys' light diet plate = Glycaemic Load = healthy weight loss (see page 92).

Glycaemic Index (GI) Foods table

Low GI	Moderate GI	High GI
Fill half your plate with these foods Asparagus, aubergine, bean sprouts, broccoli, Brussels sprouts, cabbage, cauliflower, celeriac, celery courgettes, cucumber, endive, fennel, garlic, ginger, green beans, green leafy vegetables, kale, leeks, lettuce, mushrooms, onions, peppers, radish, spinach, sprouted seeds, tomatoes, and most other vegetables which grow above the ground. Tomato soup or soup made from other vegetables listed above.	Wholewheat pasta – spaghetti is good. Rye bread and stoneground wholegrain bread. Bulgur wheat, basmati and wild rice, pitta bread, quinoa. All berries, apples, cherries, grapefruit, peaches, plums, pears, grapes, oranges, kiwi fruit, under-ripe bananas. Beans, peas and lentils. Low fat yoghurt, milk. Sweet potatoes, small new potatoes, yams, carrots, peas, broad beans, parsnips, cooked carrots, squash, swedes.	**Try to avoid these foods** White bread and croissants, bagels, pastry, white rice, breakfast cereals except porridge, biscuits, rice cakes, bread sticks, couscous. Chocolate, desserts, sweets. Higher sugar fruits (all except those listed as moderate). White potatoes (except small new). Dried fruit, and tinned fruit. Smoothies, fruit juice, soft drinks. Honey, sugar.

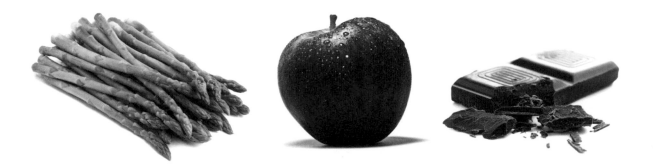

Protein: Good choices of protein include oily and white fish, eggs, skinless chicken and turkey, lean steak or ground beef, wild game meat, low fat cottage cheese and tofu.

Fats: You'll need to include some good fat at mealtimes too. Good choices include flaxseeds and oil, pumpkin, sunflower and sesame seeds, olive oil, avocado, butter, olives, plain nuts.

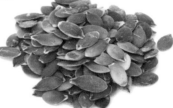

Here are some examples of how it could work:

Breakfast

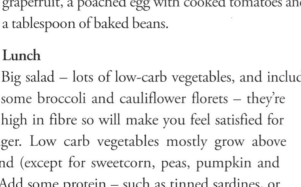

Try soaked muesli: soak 2 tbsp of porridge oats overnight in a little water and lemon juice. In the morning add some blueberries or other berries (half a cup), some walnuts (8–10), 1 tbsp flaxseeds and some plain live organic yoghurt (2–3 tbsp). Or you could have half a grapefruit, a poached egg with cooked tomatoes and a small slice of wholemeal toast or a tablespoon of baked beans.

Lunch

Big salad – lots of low-carb vegetables, and include some broccoli and cauliflower florets – they're high in fibre so will make you feel satisfied for longer. Low carb vegetables mostly grow above the ground (except for sweetcorn, peas, pumpkin and squash). Add some protein – such as tinned sardines, or eggs, or chicken breast – roughly palm sized (about 100g). Use some good fat, such as an olive oil and lemon juice dressing, or add some avocado or seeds to the salad.

Mid-afternoon

A few whole (unroasted, unsalted) almonds and an apple, or vegetable sticks and 2 tbsp of hummus.

Dinner

A portion of protein, plus plenty of low-carb vegetables, plus a modest helping of carb-rich food if you wish. Try something like salmon fillet with dill, wrapped up in an olive-oil brushed greaseproof paper parcel – securely but not tightly wrapped. Cook this in the oven at 180°C / gas mark 4 for about 20 minutes. Serve with mashed cauliflower and a mixture of steamed vegetables (leek, spinach leaves, purple-sprouting broccoli, for instance) drizzled with half a teaspoon of good olive oil. Follow this with a bowl of berries served with a tablespoon of low-fat yoghurt.

Five steps to burn fat faster

- Eat breakfast. The energy needed to digest it revs up your metabolism.

- Eat four times a day at least. Research shows that you are nearly 50% less likely to be overweight if you eat small regular meals.

- Take a supplement. CLA (conjugated linoleic acid) is a naturally occurring fatty acid with the potential to increase muscle while reducing fat storage. In an American study, 180 overweight men and women found that long-term supplementation with CLA reduced body fat – even without dieting or exercise.

- Drink green tea. Swiss research shows that drinking five cups of green tea a day increases metabolism to the extent that it could result in a weight loss of near 4 kilos a year. British research into this is also ongoing.

- Choose soya. Soya foods have been found to reduce the amount of body fat. It's thought they reduce fat storage.

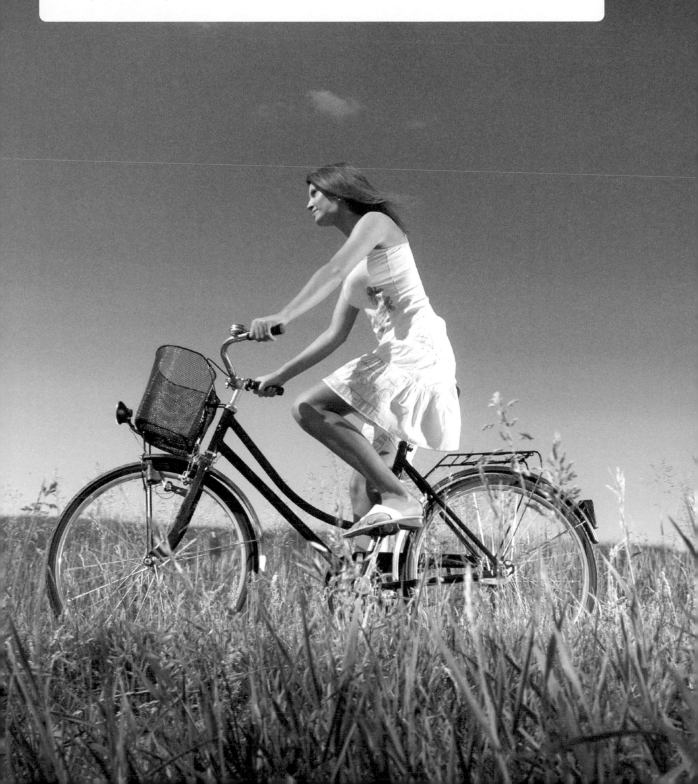

Having trouble avoiding unhealthy carbs? Get outside. Research shows that sunlight helps cut carbohydrate cravings.

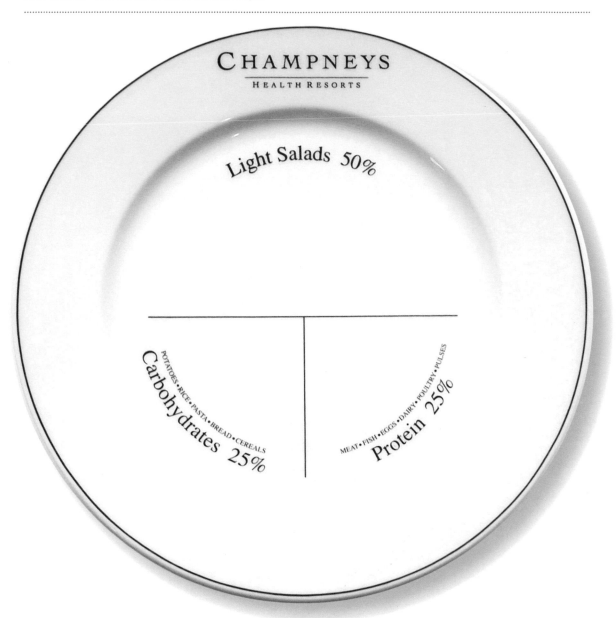

Have a picture of the light diet plate in your mind as you design your meals – coupled with the knowledge of Glycaemic Index based on the table on page 88 – and losing weight is simple. (And the big bonus is you really won't feel hungry.)

At mealtimes, you'll be filling up with lots of low-carbohydrate foods which have a low glycaemic impact, you'll eat a palm-sized portion of protein, and choose a similar amount of carb-rich food with a moderate glycaemic impact. By keeping the portion size smaller and combining it with protein, you'll control its impact on your blood sugar, how much insulin is triggered, and and how much fat you burn!

Weight loss myths

'I should be the weight on those weight and height charts…'

The charts were compiled with the assumption that excess weight was excess fat. However, if you exercise regularly, it will help you burn off excess fat and also build up lean muscle, thus boosting your metabolism. But muscle weighs more than fat, so you may not necessarily weigh a lot less although you'll look much better. This is not reflected in the charts – they make no allowance for people exercising regularly and cannot distinguish between lean muscle and fat. Minimise your use of scales and trust a mirror instead.

'I can get a flat stomach by doing 100 sit-ups a day…'

You can't spot reduce fat in a particular place. If you need to lose body fat overall, you will need to perform cardiovascular exercise to complement muscle conditioning exercises, such as abdominal curls, before the exercise will help to give you a flat stomach.

'If you eat before you exercise, you'll burn it right off…'

There is some evidence that if you exercise vigorously before you eat, you will actually eat less because of an increase in body temperature and an alteration in hormone levels (catecholamines). So it's best to avoid eating a meal before your workout; eat afterwards instead.

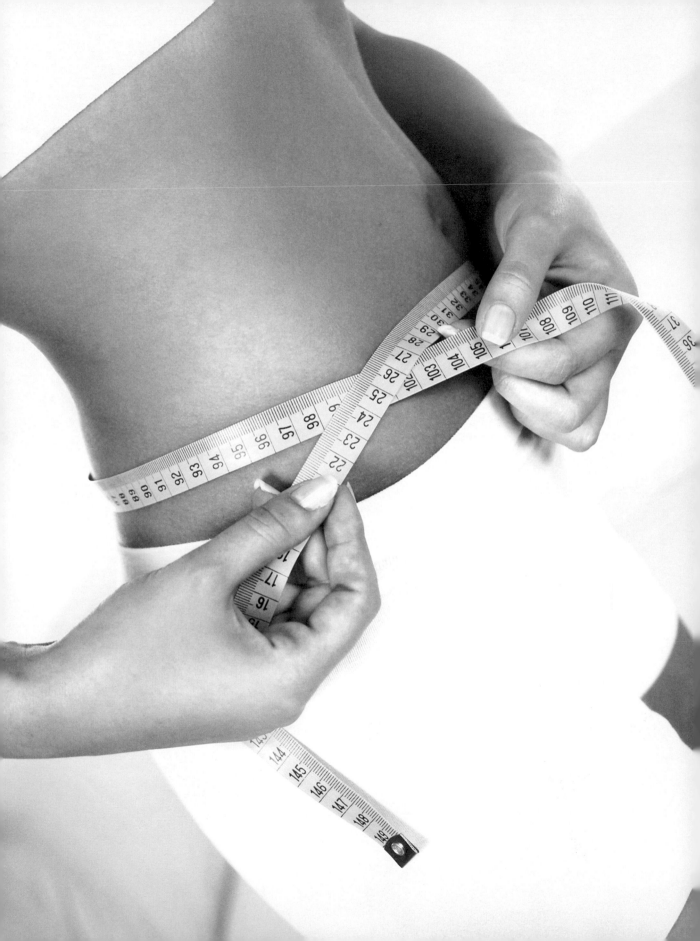

Inspiration to eat well…

Breakfasts

Champneys' fresh yoghurt muesli
(serves 4)
2 tbsp rolled oats
1 tbsp oatbran
1 tbsp wheatgerm
About 100ml skimmed milk
2 tbsp chopped mixed nuts
3 dried apricots, chopped
1 red apple, grated
1 green apple, grated
Grated zest of 1 orange
200ml low-fat Greek yoghurt
200g fresh berries
Sprigs of mint to decorate

Put the oats, oatbran and wheatgerm in a bowl, add enough milk to cover and leave to soak overnight in the fridge. In the morning, add all the remaining ingredients except the berries and the mint, and mix everything together. Stir in the berries last, then put the muesli into bowls and serve garnished with sprigs of mint.

Warm blueberry porridge
(serves 2)
250 ml skimmed or soya milk
250 ml water
100g porridge oats
A punnet of blueberries

Pour the milk and water into a saucepan and sprinkle in the oats. Bring to the boil and simmer for 4–5 minutes, stirring at all times. Remove from the heat, add the blueberries, and serve.

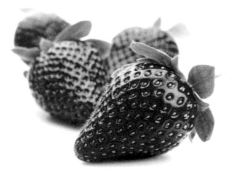

Egg white spinach omelette
(serves 1)
2 plum tomatoes, halved
1 flat mushroom
A little olive oil
50g baby spinach
Salt and pepper
3 egg whites
A scrape of butter

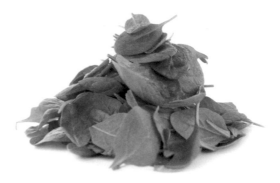

Brush the cut halves of the tomatoes and the flat side of the mushroom with a little olive oil and place them under a hot grill. Sauté the spinach in a frying pan with a little more olive oil; season with salt and freshly ground pepper. Once the spinach has wilted, drain off any excess liquid and put the spinach to one side. Pre-heat an omelette pan on the hob. Whisk the egg whites with a fork, melt a scrape of butter in the pan and add the egg whites. When they are almost cooked, place the spinach on one half and roll the other half of the omelette over it. Transfer to a plate and serve with the grilled tomatoes and mushroom.

My favourite breakfast is a small bowl of porridge. Add in a small handful of walnuts, a tablespoon of soaked linseeds, some blueberries (frozen ones are fine) and some plain live soya yoghurt. Stir and eat – delicious!

- AILSA HIGGINS, CHAMPNEYS NUTRITIONIST.

Lunches and main courses

Fresh herb soup

(serves 4)

750ml semi-skimmed milk

2 bay leaves

2 cloves

1 leek (white part only)

2 onions

2 potatoes, peeled and chopped

2 sticks of celery, sliced

2 garlic cloves, chopped

1 bunch of basil

2 tbsp low-fat fromage frais

20 green beans, blanched and finely sliced

60 broad beans, blanched and peeled

6 tbsp very finely chopped chives, chervil and parsley

Salt and pepper

Put the milk, bay leaves and cloves in a thick-bottomed saucepan and warm them over a low heat, without boiling, for about 20 minutes.

Remove the bay leaves and cloves and add the leek, onions, potatoes, celery and garlic. Bring to the simmer, cover and cook for 20–30 minutes until the vegetables are very soft. Add the basil leaves and liquidise the soup, then pass it through a sieve. Whisk in the fromage frais and then stir in the green beans, broad beans and herbs. Season to taste with salt and pepper. To serve, reheat gently without boiling.

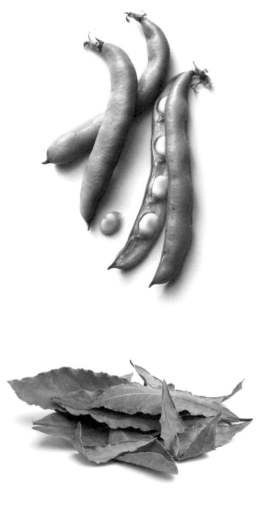

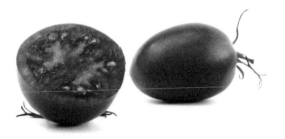

Baked plum tomato marinated in balsamic vinegar on a bed of crisp leaves with diced feta cheese

(serves 4)

4 plum tomatoes

4 tbsp balsamic vinegar

50g brown sugar

A selection of mixed leaves

450g feta cheese, diced

Pre-heat the oven to 200ºC / gas mark 6. Place the plum tomatoes on a baking tray, pour the vinegar over them and sprinkle with a little brown sugar. Bake in the oven for 10 minutes.

When they are cooked, remove them from the oven and drain off the vinegar into a small pan. Put this on a high heat, and reduce the vinegar until it has a syrupy consistency. To serve, place some mixed leaves in the middle of each plate and put the tomato on top of them. Then surround with diced feta cheese and drizzle the reduced vinegar around the edge of the plate.

Asparagus, Parma ham and mozzarella cheese

(serves 2)

8 asparagus spears

1 mozzarella ball

6 slices of Parma ham

3 tbsp olive oil, plus a little for frying

1 tbsp red wine vinegar

Chopped basil

2 handfuls of rocket leaves

Cook the trimmed asparagus and refresh it under cold water. Slice the mozzarella into two and place each half on top of two asparagus spears. Add two more spears on top and then wrap everything up in the Parma ham – each will take 2–3 slices. Warm a little olive oil in a pan and add the asparagus rolls; fry them gently until the ham is crisp and the cheese starts to melt. Whisk the 3 tablespoons of olive oil and the wine vinegar together with the chopped basil to make a dressing. Place some rocket on each plate, add the asparagus and drizzle with the dressing.

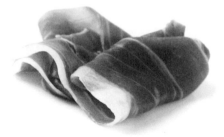

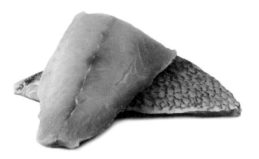

Grilled fillets of red mullet on a flat parsley, couscous and spring onion relish with a tapenade dressing

(serves 4)

4 red mullet fillets

For the relish:

1 bunch of flat parsley

6 mint leaves, shredded finely

2 tbsp couscous, soaked as per instructions on the pack

4 spring onions, finely diced

2 plum tomatoes, diced finely

Juice of 1 lemon

3 tbsp extra virgin olive oil

Salt and pepper

For the dressing:

2 tsp black olive tapenade

3 tbsp extra virgin olive oil

Black pepper

First, make the tapenade dressing. Simply mix the tapenade with the olive oil and a little black pepper, and set it aside.

Now do the relish. Mix the flat parsley, mint, couscous, spring onion and plum tomatoes in a bowl and add the lemon juice and olive oil. Season with salt and pepper. Place a shallow 8cm ring on a plate and fill it with the flat parsley relish, or simply make a neat, flat-topped pile about the same size across on each plate. Lightly grill the red mullet fillets until they are done, and place on top of the relish.

Drizzle the tepanade dressing around and serve immediately.

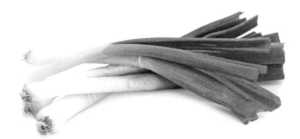

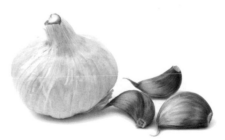

Scallop salad with avocado, mango and chilli

(serves 1)

3 scallops, shelled and cleaned

½ avocado, peeled and chopped into
    small dice

½ mango, peeled and chopped into small dice

½ red pepper, chopped into small dice

2 tsp lemon juice

1 tbsp olive oil

A few pieces of finely chopped red chilli,
    to taste

1 spring onion, chopped

Mixed leaves

Put all the ingredients, except the scallops and the mixed leaves, into a bowl and stir well to combine. Pan-fry the scallops in a little olive oil for a minute on each side. Place the scallops on a plate, add spoonfuls of the salad, and garnish with the mixed leaves.

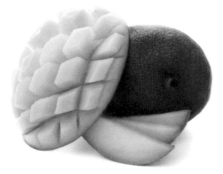

Grilled chicken with lemon and butter beans

(serves 4)

Juice of 1 lemon

2 sprigs of rosemary

1 clove of garlic, crushed

4 tbsp olive oil

Salt and pepper

4 chicken breasts, sliced in half and flattened

1 x 400g tin of butter beans, drained
    and rinsed

1 onion, finely chopped

100g rocket

Make the dressing – mix the lemon juice, rosemary and garlic with the olive oil and salt and pepper. Put the chicken in a dish and add half of the dressing; cover and leave it to marinate in the fridge for an hour. Then grill each side of the chicken for 2–3 minutes, or until it is cooked through. While the chicken is cooking, heat the beans in a pan with some fresh water, drain once warm, and add the remaining dressing, chopped onion and rocket. Place the beans on the plates and add the chicken on top. Serve immediately.

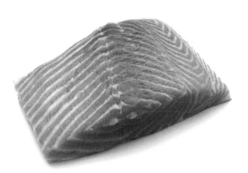

Barbecued Provençal salmon cooked en papillote

(serves 4)

8 sprigs of coriander

8 sprigs of rosemary

Juice of 1 lemon

Olive oil

225ml white wine

Salt and pepper

4 fillets of fresh salmon

2 spring onions, chopped

A small jar of sun-blushed tomatoes, chopped

A small jar of black olives, halved

1 fresh chilli, seeds removed and chopped

Mix the coriander, rosemary, lemon juice, a drizzle of olive oil, white wine and seasoning in a bowl. Put the salmon in a dish, add the herb mixture, cover and leave it to marinate for at least an hour in the fridge; overnight is even better. Place a square of tin foil approximately 50cm x 50cm on a flat surface. Put the spring onions, tomatoes and olives in the middle of the foil. Drain as much of the marinade off the salmon as possible, sprinkle it with the chilli, then place the fillets on top of the vegetables. Take hold of two of the sides of the foil and fold them together over the fish to form a sealed parcel, then scrunch the two other ends in to form a tight seal there too. Place the parcel on a thick baking tray and lay it on top of the barbecue or – if possible – just above the coals for around 15 minutes. The steam generated in the parcel will cook the salmon, help to keep it moist and allow it to take on flavours. You don't need a barbecue, though; you can bake the parcel in an oven pre-heated to 200ºC / gas mark 6 for approximately 20 minutes. Check that the salmon is cooked and, if necessary, cook a little longer. Be careful opening the parcel – the steam can be hot. Serve immediately.

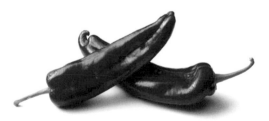

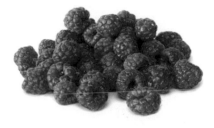

Puddings

Blue Bavarian

(serves 4)

125ml milk

3 egg yolks

50g sugar

A few drops of vanilla essence, to taste

125g fromage frais

2 tsp gelatine, dissolved according to
    packet instructions

A punnet of fresh blueberries

Bring the milk to the boil. Whisk the egg yolks, sugar and vanilla essence together in another pan. Pour the hot milk over the egg mixture, return it to heat and stir until it thickens. Remove from the heat and allow it to cool. Fold in the fromage frais and dissolved gelatine. Add the blueberries, stir together gently, and pour into four ramekins or teacups. Chill in the fridge for 2–3 hours before serving.

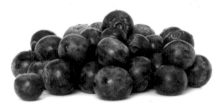

Individual raspberry and honey crème fraiche pots with an oatmeal crumble topping

(serves 4)

225g oatmeal

50g demerara sugar

225g fresh raspberries

225g low-fat crème fraiche

100g Greek yoghurt

4 tbsp clear honey

Pre-heat the oven to 180ºC / gas mark 4. Mix the oatmeal with the sugar, transfer it to an ovenproof dish and place in the oven until golden and lightly toasted – don't let it burn. Remove the dish from the oven and leave it to one side to cool.

Divide the raspberries between four ramekins, reserving four for garnishing. Whisk together the crème fraiche, Greek yoghurt and honey. Check the mixture for flavour and, if it requires more honey, add a little. Spoon the crème fraiche mixture into the ramekins leaving a space on top for the oatmeal topping. Chill them in the fridge for an hour. Remove from the fridge, place the toasted oatmeal topping on top of the ramekins and put a raspberry in the centre; serve immediately.

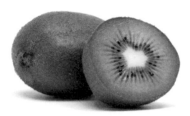

The joy of juice

Summer is a great time to buy a juicer if you haven't already done so. They are an easy way to get a whole slew of antioxidants in one hit – so mighty that regular fruit juice has been found to lower the risk of heart disease. You do miss out on the fibre of the whole food but, still, there are few things better for you on a hot day than a long drink packed with ice and a supercharged fruit or vegetable juice.

At Champneys we offer fresh fruit juices to our guests not just for their health but for the way they lift the spirit. Here are some of our guests' favourites for you to try.

The exotic
(makes a jugful)
8 kiwi fruits
5 pears
2 bananas
A punnet of strawberries
5 apples
2 litres orange juice
Put all the fruit through the juicer and top up with orange juice to taste.

Watermelon–berry granita
250g watermelon chunks, seeds removed
A punnet of fresh strawberries
(slightly overripe ones work best)
A squeeze of lemon juice
Crushed ice – as required
4 fresh mint leaves, chopped

Blend the watermelon and strawberries with a squeeze of lemon juice; strain if you wish. Then pour over crushed ice. Serve garnished with mint leaves.

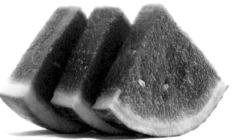

Watermelon and strawberries are high in vitamin C and vitamin B, vital for energy production and stress reduction. They also support eye health.

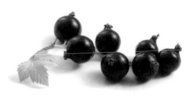

Berry booster

(serves 1)

250g low-fat yoghurt

200g mixed seasonal berries
(blueberries, blackcurrants, strawberries)

Blend these together until smooth, and serve.
(This makes a great breakfast. Add a
dessertspoon of flaxseed oil to boost your
health.)

Very special summer smoothie

(serves 4)

2 x 400g tins of peaches in natural juice

100ml Champagne

100ml crème fraiche or low-fat
natural yoghurt

Seasonal berries

Blend until smooth and garnish with fresh
berries. If this doesn't get you in the summer
mood then nothing will!

The chill-out

(makes a large jugful)

5 apples

10 carrots

A punnet of strawberries

2 litres pomegranate juice

1 litre apple juice

Put all the fruit and vegetables through the
juicer and top up with pomegranate and apple
juices to taste.

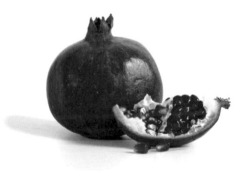

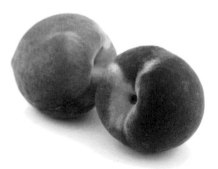

In summer, choose these seasonal foods

Strawberries, raspberries, aubergines, peas, gooseberries, broad beans, courgettes, blueberries, fennel, tomatoes, basil and greengages.

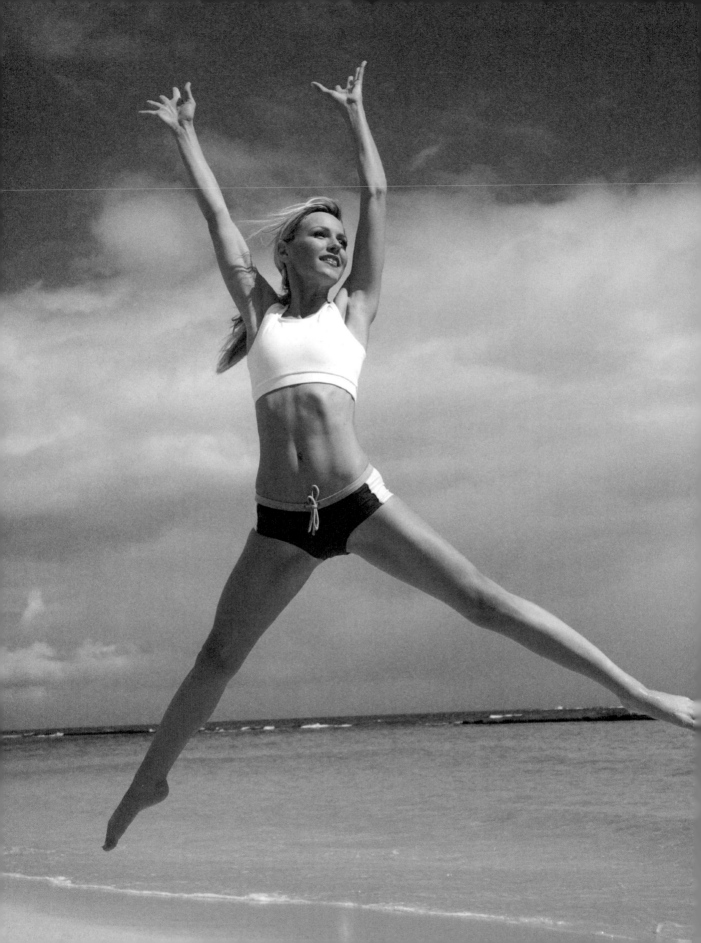

Move

'If the anti-ageing benefits of exercise came in a pill, we would go to extraordinary lengths and pay a fortune to get hold of it,' said one anti-ageing expert. So why on earth do so many of us find it hard to make exercise part of our lives? Especially when it doesn't have to be a joyless activity but a life enhancer.

Given a chance, exercise becomes as necessary as brushing your teeth and for the same reason – you don't feel right without doing it. It becomes a delight, and a way of escaping from the stress, noise and all the other problems of life.

Summer is the ideal month to begin relishing your body. Now is the time to reward it for all it does for you, and reward it with what it loves – regular, focused movement.

Do it now. Imagine that for the last week you had been exercising regularly. How would you feel now? Virtuous? Alive? Energetic? Happy to order ice cream, guilt-free? These are your motivations to exercise. Cherish them and use them as your kickstart for the following programme.

There are three main components to being fit and healthy and addressing all three should be part of your routine.

• **Cardiovascular (CV) fitness.** The better your CV fitness, the better your heart is at pumping blood around your system and the more oxygen is delivered to your tissues.

• **Muscular strength and endurance.** This is the capacity of your musculoskeletal system to exert force – in other words your ability to shift or hold weight, either free weights, weight machines or your own body. Resistance exercise builds muscle strength and endurance.

• **Flexibility.** This is the ability to stretch through a range of movements. It is important not least because it reduces the chances of suffering pain or injury as you get older.

Every element is necessary for total fitness and to age-proof your body. You may be exercising already and ready to move some new elements into your routine. You may not be exercising at all, so it may take you the whole summer to integrate all the components into a busy life. Here is how it can be done at home, but remember that there are many ways of reaching the 'fit' level other than just those we recommend. For instance, you might love Pilates and so regular classes would therefore fulfil your core strength and flexibility needs.

As usual the suggested excises assume that you are in good health. If you are pregnant or have any known health condition please consult your doctor and a qualified fitness trainer first.

If you are beginning to build your own exercise programme the most important component is cardiovascular so start with that, and add the other elements in as you go on. There are two levels of health and fitness to aim for:

- The basic health level – that's the minimum you need to do for your health;
- The fit level.

Good…
Basic health level:

- Cardiovascular: 20 minutes, three times a week – aerobic exercise;
- Muscular strength and endurance: hero conditioning moves (page 117), one set of 8–12 or 12–15 reps, twice a week – basic level;
- Flexibility: 4 hero stretches (page 123) after activity when you are warmed up, three times a week. Perform each stretch once or twice, holding for 10–30 seconds.

Better…
Fit level:

- Cardiovascular: 40–60 minutes, three to six times a week – aerobic exercise;
- Muscular strength and endurance: hero conditioning moves, (page 117), between one and three sets of 8–12 or 12–15 reps, three times a week – a more challenging weight;
- Flexibility: 8 hero stretches (page 123) after activity when you are warmed up, three times a week. Perform each stretch once or twice, holding for 10–30 seconds.

Why cardiovascular exercise is vital

Cardiovascular exercise works your heart and lungs. Keeping them strong will add years to your life and energy to those years. 'Cardiovascular' refers to any exercise that uses the big muscle groups of your body, thus increasing the demand for oxygen which they use for fuel (aerobic means using oxygen). This causes the lungs to breathe more deeply to supply this oxygen and the heart to work harder to pump the blood around your circulatory system which delivers the oxygen to your tissues. All this hard work burns excess calories by boosting your metabolism, thus maintaining a healthy level of fat in your body.

It also has a significant effect on your mood and your outlook. Cardiovascular exercise is as good as an anti-depressant in treating moderate depression, and for those of us who aren't depressed it builds a sense of optimism, self-control and a feeling of being in charge of life. It also burns off the hormones produced in response to stress which helps maintain calm.

Crucially in these hectic times, cardiovascular exercise rewards you with energy to burn. Your body becomes more efficient at using oxygen, so you don't become tired so easily. You will rise feeling rested and restored after a night's sleep. You will glide easily through your normal chores and workload and in the evening feel that you have the energy to enjoy your life rather than being frazzled and exhausted.

So cardiovascular exercise is anything that gets your heart beating faster, your lungs working harder and builds up a sweat. It includes:

Activity	Approximate calories burned per thirty minutes
Dancing	120
Walking	150
Cycling (gently)	150
Rollerblading	150
Swimming (gently)	180
Aqua aerobics	180
Tennis	210
Line dancing	240
Skiing	240
Skipping	300
Running (gently)	300
Power walking up a hill	330

You can also choose to attend aerobic classes, or buy an exercise DVD and follow it at home whenever it suits you.

How hard is enough?

If at present you do absolutely no exercise, any movement at all is better than nothing. But eventually you will want to work harder in order to get results. Getting to grips with your own 'perceived exertion scale' helps you to keep track of how effective your workouts are. For example, when you're doing shorter cardiovascular workouts, you need to focus on intensity and work harder than you would usually. That means on a perceived exertion scale of one (minimum effort) to ten (maximum, all out, effort), try to keep your intensity around what feels like seven to nine throughout the workout. It may be tough, but you may only be doing it for ten minutes.

Interval training

If you really want to strip the fat to reveal a slim, toned figure, you will need more than just regular cardiovascular exercise. Instead, try interval training. It's shorter, works better and you can use traditional cardio exercises such as cycling, walking and jogging outside. Start with a 5-minute warm up. Then you're ready for your first interval. Work hard for one minute. After 60 seconds, drop the intensity to a very easy pace for 60–120 seconds. That's one interval. Repeat the process up to 20 or 30 minutes and follow it with a cool down. You can vary the duration of the hard and easy periods – it's up to you. With interval training you'll get better results in less time than slow cardio work.

'Don't give up. Making exercise a habit is a journey, not a destination. It's something you'll work on every day...some days you'll fit it in, other days you won't. The only difference between a person who fails at regular exercise and a person who succeeds comes down to never giving up. The next time you miss a session, skip the guilt and learn from it. Become aware of your own personal and practical barriers, which get in the way of your goals and good intentions, and plan ahead in the future.'

– LOUISE DAY, CHAMPNEYS' WELL-BEING DIRECTOR AND FITNESS EXPERT

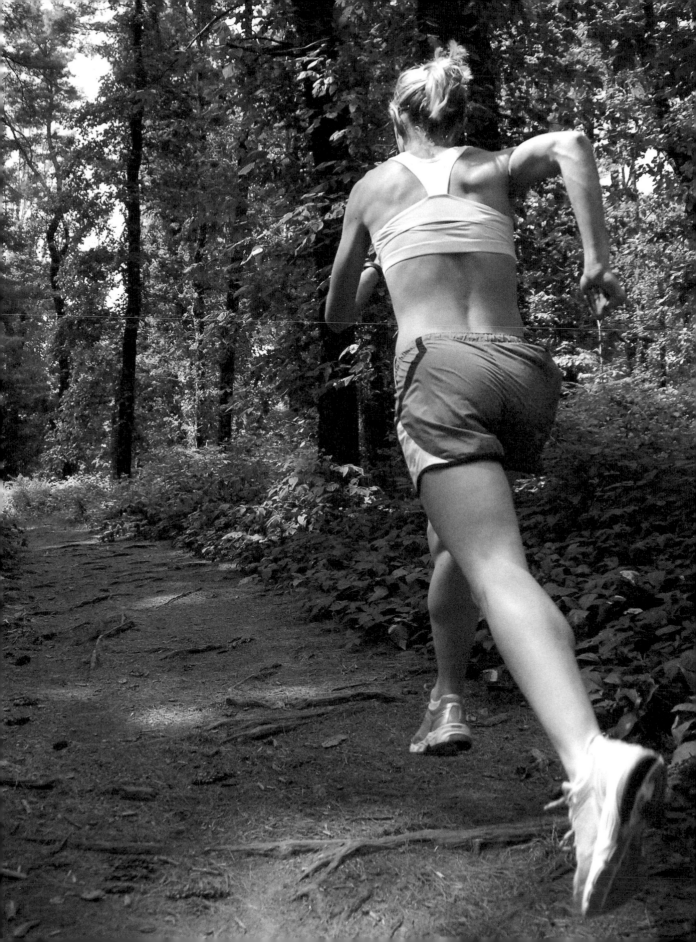

The ten-minute miracle

If you are daunted by the requirements we've given, don't panic. Research has shown that if at present you don't do much exercise you can achieve health benefits from breaking up thirty minutes a day of exercise into three ten-minute sessions, interspersed throughout the day. For instance:

- In the morning, you could spend five minutes walking briskly to the newsagent for a newspaper, then back again; walk the kids to school while they take their bikes so you have to move quickly to keep up; run up and down the stairs while you're waiting for your partner to get out of the shower!

- At lunchtime, you could power walk round the block for ten minutes or jog round the park; have lunch at a spot a bit further away than usual; walk briskly rather than dawdle round a shopping centre; do ten minutes of muscular strength and endurance or stretching exercises (see page 123).

- In the evening, you could catch up on the gardening (150 calories in ten minutes); stick on an exercise DVD and do ten minutes before you turn on your favourite programme; go for an evening walk and admire the sunset; practise some yoga before bed.

(Note that one ten-minute slot could be devoted to strength or flexibility exercise, but it's best to make two of your 10-minute sessions per day cardiovascular.)

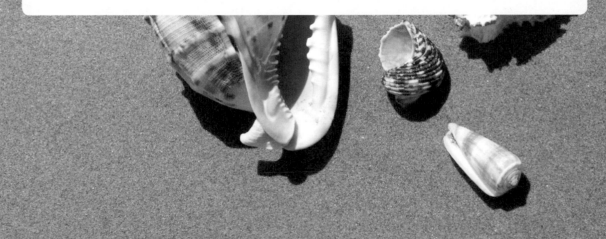

Why developing muscular strength and endurance is vital

The vast majority of people who exercise regularly (around 90% of them) lift weights as part of their regime. The reason is that it gets results fast; it builds lean muscle, which makes them look slim and burns off more energy. It stabilises joints so that they are less at risk of injury or disease. It stops muscles wasting away as they get older and thus reduces the effects of arthritis and back pain and increases bone density – particularly important for women who are more at risk of osteoporosis.

Building muscular strength and endurance through weights, Pilates, yoga or other weight-bearing exercise can transform the way your body looks and, more importantly, preserve your long-term health.

The basics

• Always warm up beforehand. You could march on the spot or step up and down stairs for 5–10 minutes and also perform mobility exercises such as shoulder rolls, knee lifts and mini squats to mobilise the joints. Then perform the stretches on page 42, the spring warm-ups, and then also at the end of the workout to reduce injury.

• A 'rep' is short for repetition and refers to a complete action from start to finish. A set is a number of reps, usually eight to twelve. The idea of weight training is that the resistance (weight) should be challenging enough to work the muscle to exhaustion within a specified number of repetitions. Each exercise is performed at a slow controlled pace and you should never compromise good posture or technique to finish a repetition. At first that might be only eight times, and from there you work up to twelve – one set. With practise and a few seconds' rest between sets, you may be able to complete two sets.

• The first weight you'll be using for some exercises is your own body. But when that becomes easy, and after a set or two you are no longer reaching muscle fatigue, you should hold weights if this is appropriate to the exercise. Then progress to heavier weights so that your workout continues to be challenging. You can use tins or bottles of water as weights to begin with, but hand-held weights are relatively inexpensive. Keep a notebook to record your number of reps and sets so that you can track your improvement.

• After exercising a group of muscles you should give them a day's rest before weight training again. So you could do your complete routine on alternate days, or work out every day but split the routine in two. However, muscles work in pairs, so work them in symmetry – if you work your chest or abdomen, do an exercise for your upper and lower back. If you work your triceps, work your biceps, too.

• Each set can take around one minute, so you really can fit weight training into even the busiest schedule.

Rediscovering your childhood grace

It's important to maintain good posture when exercising, including throughout your weight training session. When standing, feet should be hip distance apart, planted firmly on the ground, knees never locked but 'soft' and shoulders naturally relaxed and away from your ears. Probably most important of all you should maintain what fitness experts call 'neutral spine'. In other words, your back should show the beautifully elegant curves that you adopted effortlessly in childhood.

Try this

Stand as above and draw your navel towards your spine. Ensure that you look straight ahead, chin parallel to the floor and feel as if the top of your head is attached to a piece of string that is pulling it away from your body, lengthening out your neck and spine. Now place the thumbs of each hand at the bottom ribs and the first fingers underneath them on the hip bones. Tilt the pelvis, without moving the upper body, allowing the lower back to flatten and the bottom to tuck under. You will feel the fingers and thumb coming closer together. Now using the abdominal muscles bring the pelvis back to the centre. Tilt the pelvis the opposite way allowing the bottom to stick out and your tummy to protrude: feel the distance between the fingers and thumb increase. Now find the half way position between the two extremes. This is neutral spine i.e. the spine maintaining its natural curves.

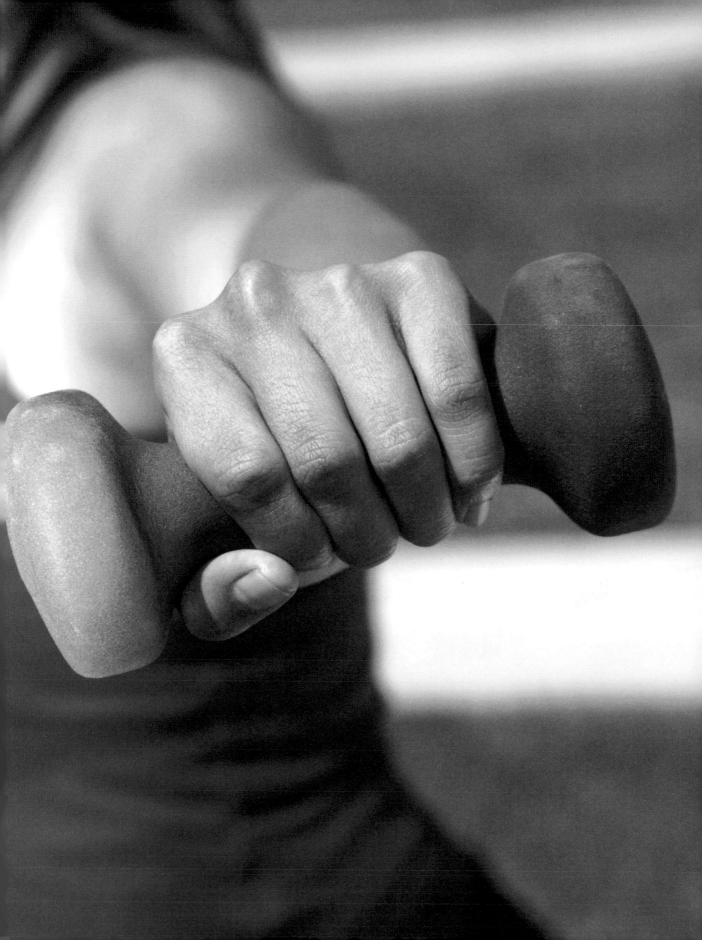

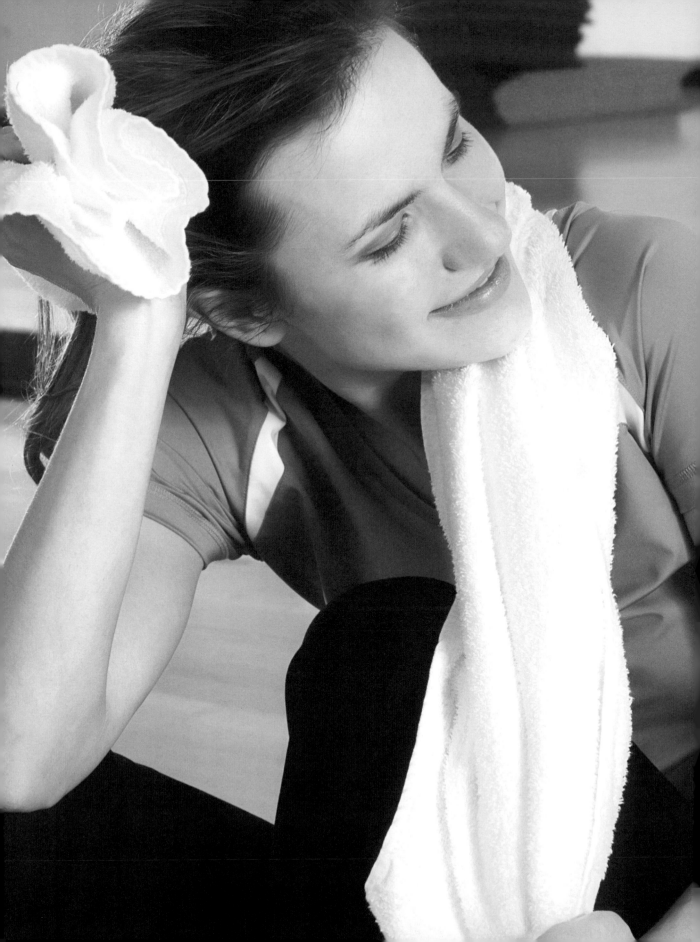

Champneys' eight hero moves

At Champneys we teach these muscular strength and endurance exercises first – the 'hero whole body conditioning moves' that will show results fast and are functional to everyday life.

Squats – to tone the legs

Place your feet slightly wider than shoulder width apart, toes pointed forward or slightly out. From neutral spine, lean forwards from the hips, push your buttocks out behind and squat until your knees are near 90 degrees. Ensure that your weight is in the heels and that your knees stay behind your toes. Try to imagine you were going to sit in a chair, but as your bottom gets level with your knees, you change your mind. Rise from the squat position to standing by bringing the hips back in alignment and keeping your chest lifted. Keep your navel in to support the lower back throughout the exercise.

Option: arms reach forward as you squat.

Next: build up to holding weights.

Lunges – to tone the legs

Stand tall, with your feet approximately hip width apart. Keeping one foot where it is, take a large step back and bend the knees. Control the descent, don't just drop, bringing your front thigh parallel to the floor. Your front knee should remain above the ankle and keep the back heel lifted. Push off the rear leg and return back to the start position. Keep alternating sides.

Keep your stomach pulled in and your shoulders pulled back. Option: To make it easier hold on to a chair for balance with one hand.

Next: build up to holding weights, or even try stepping forwards or out to the sides which relate to various positions you'll move in during the course of the day.

Press-ups – to tone the chest and arms

Kneel on the floor placing your hands shoulder width apart in line with your shoulders. Place your knees hip distance apart, in line with the hips. Maintain neutral spine and draw your navel in towards your spine. Bend at the elbows, lowering your chest to the floor until your elbows are at ninety degrees but stopping at a fist's distance from it. Push back up without locking the elbows.

Next: kneel on the floor, with your knees together and take your body weight forward onto the fleshy part of the knee above the kneecap, crossing your ankles and raising them off the floor. Place your hands shoulder width apart, in line with your shoulders. Repeat excercise as above.

Single arm row
– to tone the upper back and arms

Place your left hand with elbow extended (but not locked) and the left knee on a flat bench. Keep your shoulders parallel to the floor maintaining neutral spine and navel to spine throughout. Holding a weight directly under the shoulder in your right hand, lift the elbow towards the ceiling, keeping the weight close to the body. Keep your upper half as still as possible. Slowly lower the weight back to the start position. After one set, repeat on the other side.

Next: use heavier weights.

Abdominal curls – to tone the abdominals

Lie on your back with your knees bent and feet hip distance apart. Find neutral spine, breathe in and, as you breathe out, draw your navel towards your spine. Place both hands on your thighs. Now slowly slide your hands up the thighs towards your knees letting your head and shoulders curl up off the floor as they get higher. Keep your chin off your chest and slowly roll back. Breathe out as you lift, breathe in as you lower. Remember that height is not important. Instead, focus on scooping in the abdominals throughout the exercise.

Next: do as above but cross your arms over your chest and then progress to keeping your hands either side of your head with the elbows back.

Back extensions
– to strengthen the back

Lie face down on the floor with your elbows positioned at right angles so that they are in line with the shoulders, palms flat and shoulders down and relaxed. Draw your navel towards your spine and lift the chest and head slowly from the floor, keeping your neck in line with the spine by looking down to the floor. Your forearms and hands should remain in contact with the floor. Aim not to lift your upper body far from the floor as this is essentially a long, low stretch.

Next: As above but with arms by your sides.

Tricep dips – to tone the back of the upper arms

Sit upright on a bench, placing one hand either side of the hips. Walk your feet out until your bottom comes away from the bench. Place your feet at hip distance, with knees in line with your ankles. Bend your elbows and lower your body weight down until the elbows form a 90 degree angle at the joint, pointing directly behind you. Return back to the starting position. Throughout the exercise keep your back close to the bench and pull your navel towards your spine.

Next: walk your feet out so the legs are straight and repeat the exercise above.

Bicep curls – to tone the front of the upper arms

Stand with your feet hip distance apart, knees soft and keep neutral spine. Grasp the weights with an underhand grip and hold them at your thighs. Lift the weights up to the shoulders, keeping your elbows close to the sides of the body throughout the exercise. Keep your shoulders down and relaxed, navel to spine.

Next: build up to heavier weights.

Especially if you are a beginner it is a good idea to seek the advice of a fitness trainer to ensure your form is safe and correct.

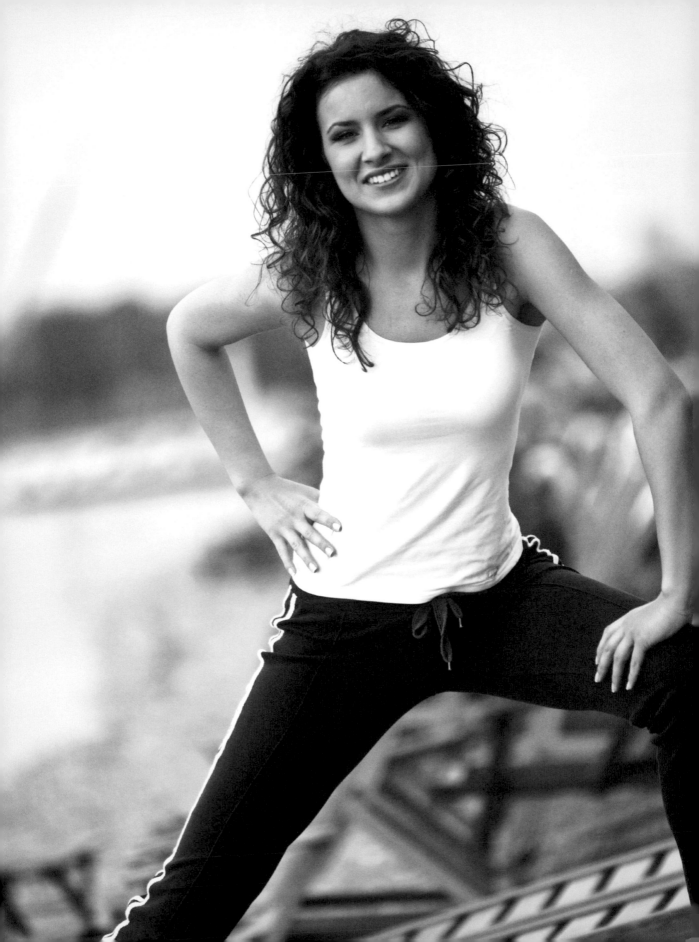

Why developing flexibility is vital

Being flexible makes life simpler. When you can reach easily for the book on the top shelf, bend effortlessly to retrieve a dropped ball, join in the rough and tumble with the kids without fearing you'll 'do' your back in, life is more enjoyable. You are less stressed, you hold less tension in your neck and shoulders – and if you do feel that life is getting on top of you, all you need is a few moments and some simple movements and the kinks are ironed out.

If you do this, you will have increased joint mobility and be less at risk of back pain and other chronic disabilities. These exercises also have the added benefit of conveying a sense of calm and spirituality to your everyday life.

You will have more presence, walk taller, command more attention without opening your mouth – flexibility exercise improves posture and boosts self-esteem. It's amazing the difference that lifting back your shoulders and looking the world in the eye can make to your sense of self. Follow the guidelines below:

• If you feel like a stretch to relax you (and it does become swiftly both addictive and alluring at any time of day or evening), remember to always warm up beforehand. You could march on the spot or step up and down stairs for 5–10 minutes and perform mobility exercises like shoulder rolls, knee lifts and mini squats to mobilise the joints before performing the stretches on page 123.

• Concentrate on the muscles you are stretching and work towards feeling the stretch in the middle of the muscle you are working on. Be slow and focused. Movement should be measured.

• Perform each stretch once or twice. Hold each stretch for around ten to thirty seconds. Breathe naturally and try to relax into the stretch and hold it until it is slightly uncomfortable. Never push on if the stretch is painful or bounce in and out of the stretch.

• Always maintain good posture.

• If you wish, play some calming music to help you relax.

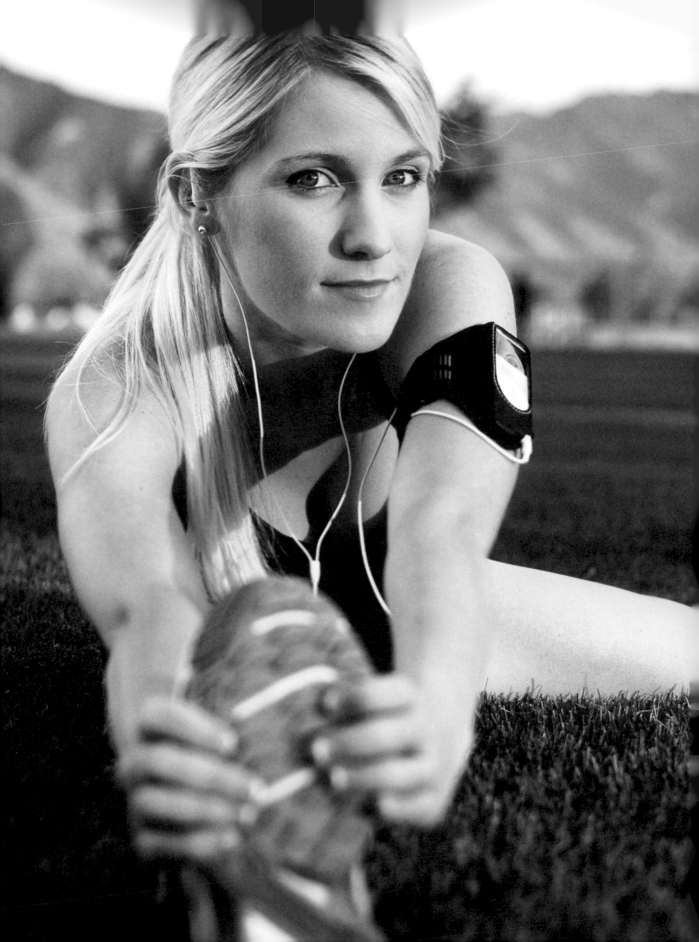

Champneys' twelve hero stretches

Here are the stretches that form our basic flexibility routine. As you become more confident you may wish to extend your programme, hold each stretch a few seconds longer or try alternative stretches to develop your flexibility. Yoga, Pilates and T'ai Chi also help to improve flexibility and you may want to experiment with those, too, mixing some of those postures into your routine.

Neck stretch

In a standing position, with neutral spine and navel to spine, draw the shoulder blades down the back and tilt the head to one side whilst looking forward. Repeat on the other side.

Shoulder stretch

In a standing position, with neutral spine and navel to spine, hold your left arm ahead of you and grasp it just below the left elbow with the right hand. Gently pull it across to the right shoulder. Do not twist the upper body or turn your shoulders or hips. Repeat with the right arm.

Upper back stretch

In a standing position, with neutral spine and navel to spine, clasp your hands in front of you and raise them upwards until they are at shoulder height. Drop your head slightly and round the upper body, pulling your shoulder blades gently away from each other. Avoid locking your elbows.

Chest stretch

In a standing position, clasp your hands behind your back and raise them upwards, opening out the chest. Avoid locking the elbows. Maintain neutral spine, and pull your navel in towards your spine.

Backs of upper arms

In a standing position, raise one arm above the head and place your hand between your shoulder blades. Use the other hand to gently press the arm back, keeping the arm close to the ear. Repeat with the other arm. Keep your head up, maintain neutral spine and pull your navel in towards your spine.

Back of the thigh

Sit with the sole of one foot resting on the inner thigh of the other leg. Turn the upper body to face the outstretched leg. Sit up tall and lean forwards from the hips until you feel a comfortable, mild stretch in the back of your thigh. Avoid rounding your back in an attempt to get your nose on your knee! Maintain a neutral spine. Place your hands either side of the leg. Repeat with the other leg.

Inner thigh stretch

Sit tall with the soles of the feet together and hold on to your ankles so your legs form a diamond shape. Relax your legs in this position and, after several seconds, gently press your knees towards the floor with your elbows. Hold the stretch.

Calf stretch

Sit tall and either use a towel around the ball of your foot to gently pull your foot towards your knee or, if you are more flexible, use your hands to draw your foot towards your knee. Find a mild, comfortable stretch and hold. Repeat on the other side.

Front of thigh

Lie on your front, resting your head on one hand. Bend the knee of the opposite leg, taking hold of the foot, and ease it towards your buttocks. Keep your knees together, maintaining a small gap between your heel and bottom. Gently press your hips into the floor. If this position is difficult, hold on to the ends of a towel wrapped around your ankle. Repeat on the other side maintaining good body alignment.

Back stretch

Lie on your back, knees to chest. Holding your legs behind your thighs, ease the legs down towards your chest, allowing the buttocks to rise slightly from the floor. Separate your knees if it helps.

If you prefer, adopt the 'all fours' position, placing your hands underneath your shoulders and knees underneath hips; your elbows should be soft. Gently pull upwards, arching your back while dropping your head in towards the chest.

Hip flexor stretch (front of hip)

Kneel down on one knee and take a big step forward with the other leg. Squeeze the buttocks on the side being stretched and gently press the hips forward until you feel a mild comfortable

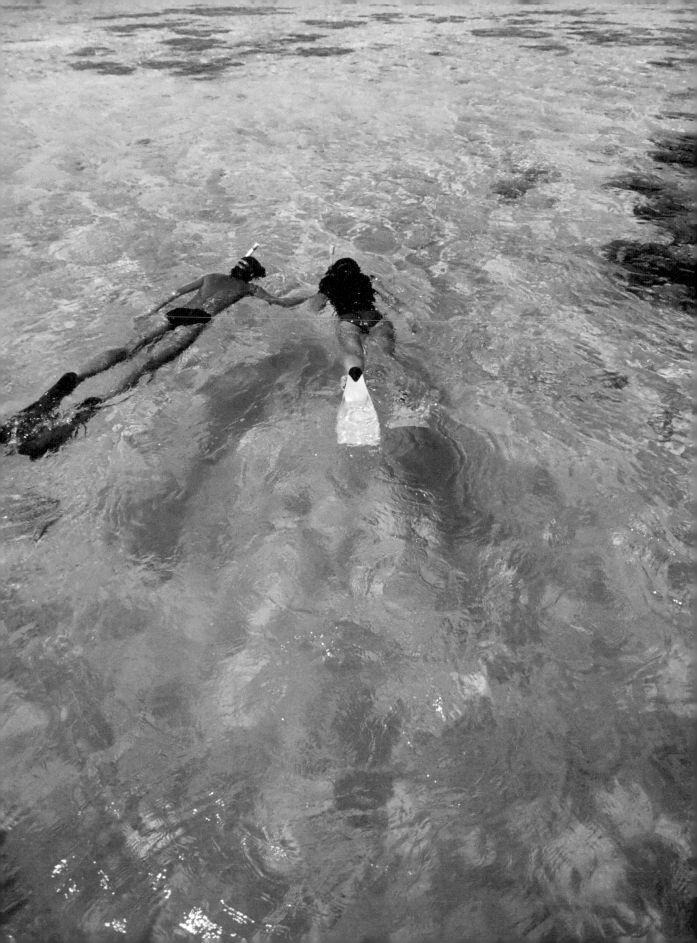

stretch in the hip area. The front knee should be bent at right angles i.e. with your knee in line with your ankle. Hold for a minimum of twenty seconds and then repeat the stretch on the opposite leg behind the toes.

Option: Kneel on a towel or cushion for comfort if required.

Outer hips and buttocks

Lie on your back with both knees bent and feet on the floor. Now cross an ankle over the opposite knee and allow the knee and hip to relax and open out. Increase the stretch by lifting the other foot off the floor, taking hold of that leg behind the thigh and easing it towards your chest. Repeat on the other side.

The relaxation routine

Elongation stretch

Lie on your back and extend your arms overhead and stretch your legs straight out. Now reach your arms and legs as far as is comfortable in the opposite direction. Stretch for five seconds and then relax.

Diagonal stretch

Now stretch diagonally. Point the toes of your left foot as you extend your right arm above your head. Hold five seconds and then relax. Stretch your right leg and left arm in the same way. Hold the stretch for five seconds, then relax.

…and completely relax

Now let your feet fall outwards with your arms relaxed beside your body with the palms up. Regulate your breathing and enjoy a few minutes of total rest. Cover yourself with a blanket if it makes you feel more secure and comfortable.

Now put it all together with our 'Be Active' programme…

The easiest ever holiday workout

Just as you get into the routine of exercising regularly, your summer holiday rolls around and the good habits are broken. But not this year. The principle of the ten-minute miracle (page 112) will allow you to keep fit with minimal effort…

- **Water walking for ten minutes.** At waist-level, wade across the breadth of the pool (or through the sea) at a slow pace for four widths and then as fast as you can for four widths, then two slow, four fast for a total of ten minutes.

- **Swimming for ten minutes.** Stay motivated by increasing the number of lengths, reducing the number of strokes per length and/or aiming for faster times.

- **Beach strolling for ten minutes**. Walking on fine sand in bare feet uses two and half times more energy than walking on grass.

- **Strength training in your hotel room for ten minutes.** Tricep dips can be done against your bed or a sturdy chair. Lunges, squats, press-ups, abdominal curls and back extensions don't require any equipment. Two bottles of water can double up as weights for single arm rowing and bicep curls. And there you have it, a complete balanced workout.

You should be feeling more active this summer after your new programme of body and exercise awareness. Get in the pool with the kids, play table tennis, go for a hike as the day cools down, play beach volleyball or cricket. Don't refuse an invitation to be active and you'll be amazed at your energy levels.

It takes around six weeks to form a new habit. It will make it easier to stick at the Be Active programme if you reward yourself with a sensual body treat every time you complete your workout.

Escape – Be active

The Champneys Be Active programme is designed to help people form the exercise habit. You can try it at home with the following plan.

If you are a beginner, or a sporadic exerciser, start with the basic health level and work up to the fit level. Here's a reminder:

Basic health level:

Cardiovascular: 20 minutes, three times a week – aerobic exercise

Muscular strength and endurance: hero conditioning moves (page 117), one set of 8–12 or 12–15 reps twice a week – basic level

Flexibility: 4 hero stretches (page 123) after activity when you are warmed up, three times a week. Perform each stretch once or twice, holding for 10–30 seconds

Fit level:

Cardiovascular: 40–60 minutes, three to six times a week – aerobic exercise

Muscular strength and endurance: hero conditioning moves (page 117), between one and three sets of 8–12 or 12–15 reps, three times a week – a more challenging weight

Flexibility: 8 hero stretches (page 123) after activity when you are warmed up, three times a week. Perform each stretch once or twice, holding for 10–30 seconds

See how easy it can be to fit this into your week, bearing in mind that the flexibility exercises take a few minutes, the muscular strength and endurance ones around ten minutes and cardiovascular ones from twenty minutes…

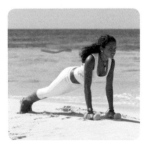

Monday Muscular strength and endurance hero moves or other resistance training exercise such as Pilates or a fitness DVD.

Tuesday Cardiovascular exercise followed by flexibility session; hero stretches or yoga.

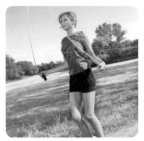

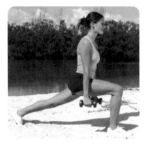

Wednesday Muscular strength and endurance hero moves or other resistance training.

Thursday Cardiovascular exercise followed by flexibility session; hero stretches or yoga.

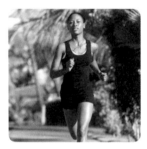

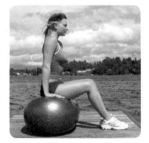

Friday Muscular strength and endurance hero moves or other resistance training exercise.

Saturday Cardiovascular exercise followed by flexibility session; hero stretches or yoga.

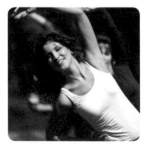

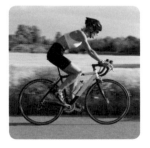

Sunday Rest or a walk in the country, a yoga class or bike ride – anything as long as it's fun.

What's holding you back?

If you have started numerous exercise routines but never been able to stick at any of them, could there be reasons other than your lack of motivation? Pick the answer that best describes you.

Where is your recent gas bill?

a) no idea – maybe at the bottom of your handbag, maybe stuck on the fridge.

b) it's on direct debit. You're way too busy to deal with bills.

c) it's waiting to be paid, with the rest of the bills you haven't got round to yet.

You are late to meet an old friend, she will…

a) assume that you've got the date wrong.

b) assume you've been held up by another crisis at work – again.

c) assume that you are on your way but late because you nearly always are a little late.

You see an ad for a job you might like but…

a) it's such a hassle updating your CV and getting the application together. And you can't remember where you filed the ad in the first place.

b) you can't see how you'll find three hours to sit down and do an application – you're just too busy.

c) you hope there's plenty of time to apply. You need to spend hours getting your CV right and thinking about how to present yourself.

Now turn the page to see how you did and find out how to improve your motivation.

Mostly **a**? You may simply be too disorganised to exercise. You seem to take life as it comes to you, without doing much planning. Developing an exercise routine takes a certain amount of forward thought – you have to carve out the time. See Louise's first tip below.

Mostly **b**? You live a hectic life, which you enjoy. But it means that exercise gets shunted to the side when another 'fire' that must be put out arises. Exercise will help you manage stress. See Louise's fourth tip below.

Mostly **c**? Exercise may be another thing you keep putting off. Procrastinators are often perfectionists. Remember, you don't need to start off with a perfect routine, just start with ten minutes a day. And if that's too much, see Louise's fifth tip below.

Motivation guaranteed

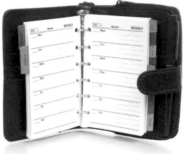

Louise Day, Champneys' fitness expert, believes that those who keep to the guidelines below will find it easier to stick to an exercise programme.

1. Commit – when you fail to plan you plan to fail. To be successful, pencil in an exact appointment and consider it as you would a business meeting.

2. Break it up – exercise does not have to be carried out in one session. You can split your exercise time in two by doing some exercise in the morning before work, then more later in the day. Research suggests that the fitness benefits of segmented exercise may be as great as one longer effort.

3. Recruit a friend, join a class or book a personal trainer for support.

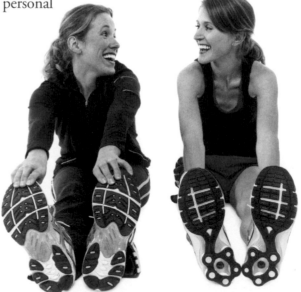

4. Utilise the weekend – your schedule is more flexible then and under your control.

5. See your life as a workout. Go up the stairs as often as possible. For variety, take the stairs two at a time, or step up the pace. When you park the car, look for the longest rather than the shortest route. Get up from your chair (permanently lose the TV remote). When unloading groceries from your car, carry one bag at a time into the house. View chores like lawn mowing, dusting and vacuuming as opportunities to exercise – and go for it with purpose.

6. Vary and enjoy your exercise. If you don't enjoy what you have chosen to do you will not continue to do it. You should also change what you do every so often. An exercise programme should range between 3 and 12 weeks, which is the amount of time your body needs to adapt to new training and make physical improvements. After this period, your gains will level off because, basically, you have become better at this given exercise plan. Change duration, intensity (e.g. interval training), mode of exercise or even consider changing the order of exercises. This will keep you motivated.

7. Be realistic. Base your goals for change on facts rather than ideals. Setting simple, attainable goals keeps your motivation high. If you can only get to an exercise class three times a week realistically – don't set yourself the target of five times a week. Remember instant results are something that we all crave but there are no quick fixes when it comes to getting and staying in shape.

Cellulite solutions

Exercise is one of the most effective and inexpensive ways to smooth out those unwanted cellulite lumps and bumps. Any exercise should help reduce and prevent the appearance of more cellulite, and the more regular and often you work out, the better.

Exercise is effective in helping reduce cellulite on a number of levels. Exercise burns many more calories compared to sitting still, and even after exercise the body continues burning calories at an increased rate for up to twelve hours. As well as losing fat you also gain muscle mass, which in turn causes the body to burn more calories. Muscle is a metabolically active tissue so the more it is used the more calories are burned. Muscle can also make cellulite less noticeable as it stops the fibres of collagen that run through fat cells pulling down on the skin.

Exercise helps stimulate circulation, too. It also helps boost the lymph flow which, unlike circulation, does not have a pump to propel it around the body. Instead it relies on the contraction of muscles to push it along. This action is intensified when you exercise.

Even though any exercise can help reduce the appearance of cellulite, not all exercise works in the same way so it is beneficial to use a combination of different types. Try to do at least twenty minutes every day of either cardio or muscular strength and endurance exercises.

A top move to help reduce the appearance of cellulite

In addition to squats and lunges, this is a good exercise for smoothing the thighs. Stand as if you were about to do a traditional plié, with your legs wider than shoulder width apart, toes pointed out slightly, hands on hips. Bend your knees, lowering until your thighs are almost parallel with the floor. Keep your spine neutral and your tummy muscles held in. Hold the position for the count of three. Stand up and swing your right leg forward and to the left as if you were about to kick a ball across the body, but keep your foot flexed and hips facing the front. Return to the start position.

Do ten reps with the right leg and then swap to the left leg and repeat. Work up to three sets of fifteen reps with each leg, and do it three times a week.

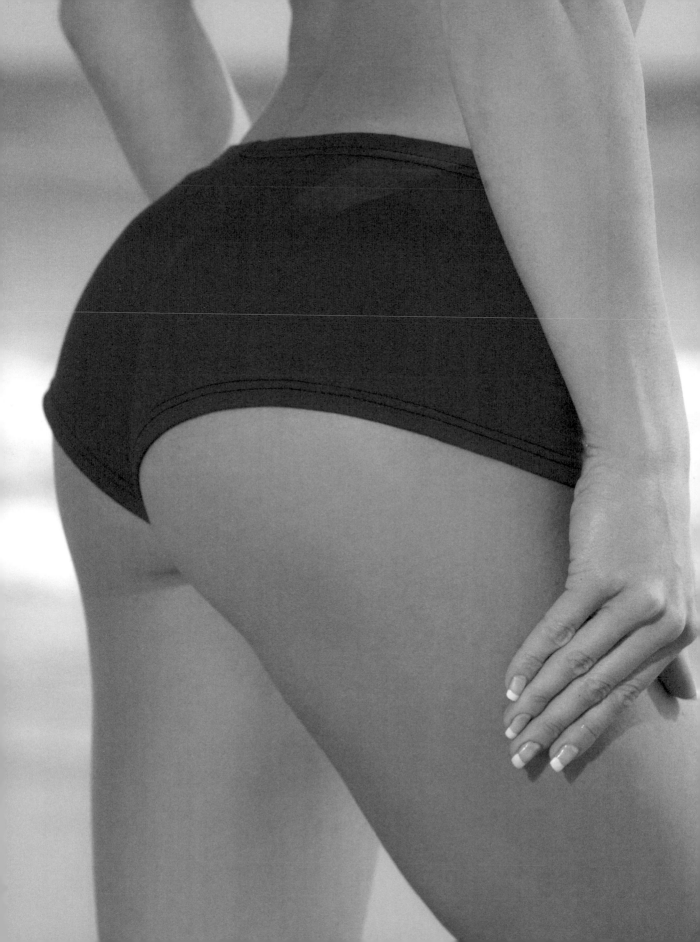

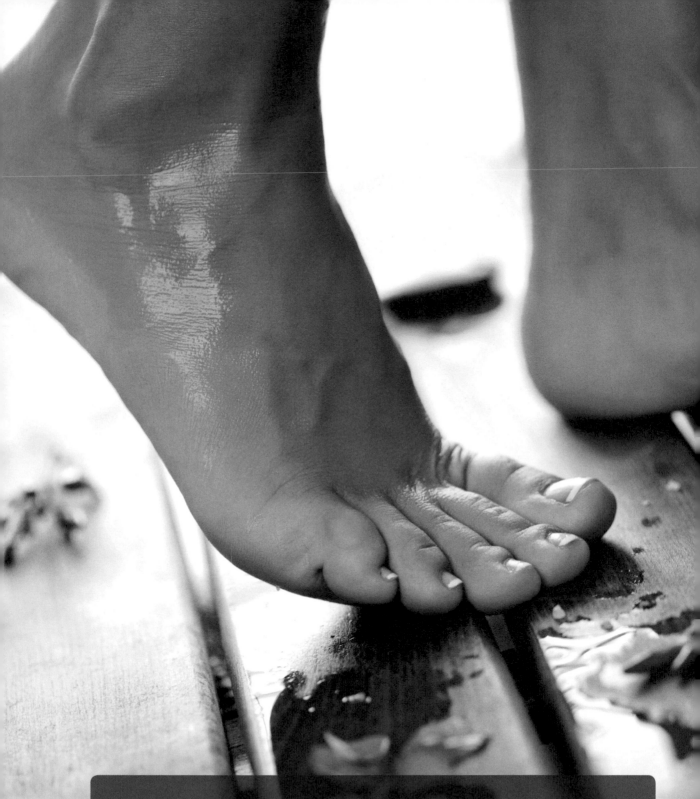

Summer is a time for lavishing attention on the parts of your body, such as your feet, that don't usually get enough love and care.

Love yourself

The Hip and Thigh Detoxifier

This localised treatment specifically targets areas that are prone to cellulite. A combination of body brushing and exfoliating techniques are combined with a drainage massage resulting in your legs feeling firm, smooth and toned.

You'll need a body brush, mitts, a towel and a good quality massage oil such as Champneys Firm and Tone Aromatherapy Oil. A great investment for this treatment is Champneys Deep Tissue Toning Massager, an electric massager that gives a salon level of stimulating massage and will really help shift cellulite.

Before you start use Champneys Firm and Tone Aromatherapy Oil or make your own anti-cellulite oil by adding 20 drops of juniper oil, 10 drops of cypress and 10 drops of rosemary oil to 25ml of carrier oil.

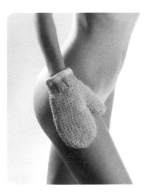

Body brushing
Start with the left leg at the ankle, body brush to the knee and then, using a firm stroke, massage with the hand. Brush then stroke the thigh, moving upward. Repeat on the right leg.

Exfoliate
Step into the shower and use an exfoliater, such as Champneys Aqua Therapy Refining Salt Scrub, to exfoliate your legs. Start with left, then right. Shower off the exfoliater and dry your legs.

Massage
With firm, sweeping strokes apply Champneys Firm and Tone Aromatherapy Oil or your own anti-cellulite oil from your ankles to the top of your thighs.

Massage with the Deep Tissue Toning Massager (or with your hands) using firm strokes and working from the ankles over the lower leg and then the thigh, left leg first. Use both hands to knead into the skin. Spend five minutes working on each thigh, really working at a deep level.

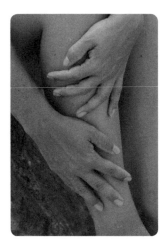

After kneading, use firm, sweeping strokes from ankle to knee six times and then from knee to thigh six times, on your left and then right leg.

Apply body lotion, such as Champneys Aqua therapy Moisture Rich Firming Lotion all over your legs.

Sit with your legs lightly bent at the knee. Then, using the thumbs and circular movements, work along the side of the calf of your left leg. Work from the ankle to the back of the knee and return. Concentrate on the centre of the calf; crossing your thumbs, apply medium pressure from the ankle to the back of the knee and glide back to the ankle.

Start at the ankle with your fingers enveloping the calf, and squeeze the full length of the calf. When your fingers hit the diamond at the back of the knee, press with your thumbs and then glide back to the ankle. Repeat on the right leg. Apply body lotion again.

Wrap and rest

Now cover your legs with a blanket and relax on your bed with your legs elevated using a cushion under your calves. Stay there for as long as you can.

Unleash your sensuality

Summer is the time for revelling in the sensual side of life. How many of these have you done in the last fortnight?

- Massaged your skin with scented lotion. ☐
- Walked into a room, thinking 'I look terrific'. ☐
- Bathed by candlelight. ☐
- Got totally caught up in a song and sung along. ☐
- Made the first move. ☐
- Laughed so hard you probably didn't look pretty. ☐
- Worn a fabric that made you feel good all day. ☐
- Watched a sunset or sunrise. ☐
- Danced anywhere – your kitchen counts… ☐
- Bought a beauty product that you didn't really need. ☐

If you ticked three or fewer, open your mind, heart and body to the endless sensual pleasure available to you. You'll feel happier – and more confident.

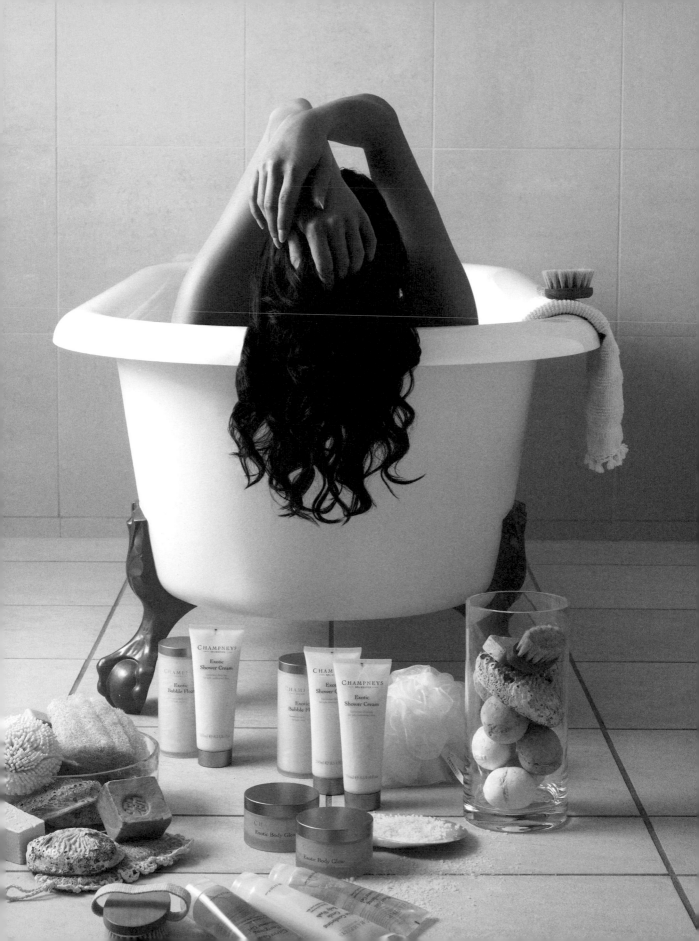

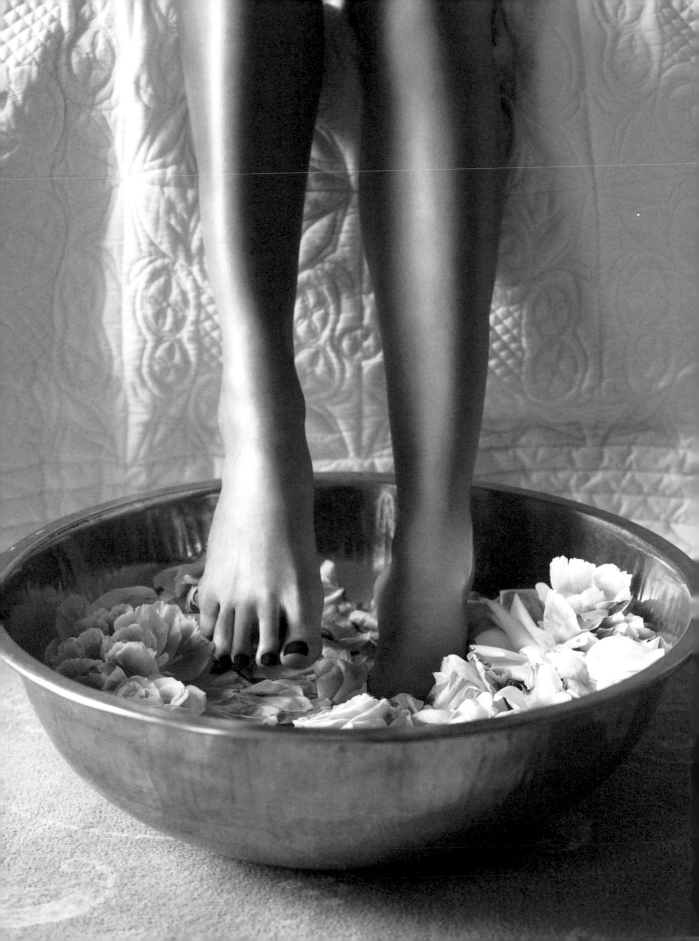

Sensual luxury foot massage

This is a deeply grounding treatment that will calm you down at any point of the day. (Try it on children; it works on them, too.)

Before you start: find a quiet spot, perhaps under a shady tree. You will need an intensive moisturiser and a towel or soft socks.

Massage

- Apply an intensive moisturiser such as Champneys Deeply Moisturising Softening Foot Butter or Intensive Cracked Heel Treatment Balm.

- Use both hands to envelop and massage the left foot, six times.

- Use the fingers of both hands to circle the ankles and rotate, six times.

- With both thumbs, apply friction all round the ankles six times.

- With both thumbs, apply friction to the top of the foot six times.

- Starting at your big toe, work towards the little toe pressing on the top of each toe, six times.

- From pad to heel, work down the sole pressing and releasing six times.

- Circle the sole from pad to heel in large circles, six times.

- Use your fist to knuckle the sole; support your foot with other hand.

- Squeeze each foot with your thumbs, working from heel to toes, six times.

- Give a firm pull to each toe.

- Repeat for your right foot.

Wrap and rest

Now slather on moisturiser and wrap a towel around your feet or pop on some cotton socks. Lie back with your feet elevated. Having warm feet is grounding and relaxing at an almost primal level.

Peace of mind

Get outside as much as you can (making sure you wear sun lotion, of course). Being under the open sky relaxes us on a deep level.

- Lie on the grass and practise the meditation technique of the body scan. Focus on your breathing and begin to scan your body. Bring your attention to tense areas and 'breathe into them'; exhale the tension. Start from the head to toe, or the other way around. This is a good way of becoming more aware of your body and, with practice, you will find you live less in your head and are more in touch with the sensual side of life.

- Enjoy an outdoor massage… treat yourself on the beach, under a tree, in any shady corner. It's much more relaxing in the open air.

- Eat al fresco whenever the weather allows. Even just ten minutes drinking a cup of tea in the garden will relax you for the rest of the day.

Express pedicure

You'll need a cuticle stick, nail file, buffing block, nail clippers, foot file, oil such as Champneys Nail and Cuticle Wonder Oil.

Before you start prepare a summer foot soak. Fill a bowl large enough for your feet with warm water. Add a handful of freshly torn mint, and ten drops of tea tree essential oil. Place the bowl near your favourite relaxing spot and cue up some quiet music.

- Remove any polish from your toenails.
- Remove hard skin with the foot file.
- Soak your feet for ten minutes in the summer foot soak.
- Push back the cuticles using the cuticle stick.
- Apply one drop of oil per nail and massage it in.
- Cut and file your nails.
- Apply moisturiser (or undertake the entire summer foot massage as a special treat).
- Use nail polish remover to remove any excess product from the nails.
- Use tissues or a toe separator to allow more effective toenail painting.
- Now for the nail colour. Apply one base coat, two coats of colour and a single layer of top coat.
- When the varnish is completely dry, massage in one drop of oil per nail, concentrating on the cuticle only.

Fresh Face Facial

This is a refreshing, deep-cleansing facial to polish away dull, patchy skin, revealing a fresh-face ready for minimal summer make-up – and facial self-tanning products, if you use them.

The Champneys' face cleanse routine which is described here can be used on a daily basis to ensure a proper cleanse and to stimulate skin cells. You can also use a complexion brush every few days and adapt the routine accordingly when you require extra exfoliation. To perform the facial you could use a professional tool such as Champneys Fresh Face Micro-Dermabrasion System.

Before you start remove eye make-up with eye make-up remover and, using Champneys Skin Comforting Gentle Cleansing Milk or your usual cleanser, get rid of superficial lip and face make-up ready for a deep cleanse.

Deep cleanse by using a small amount (roughly 2 cm or the size of a 10p piece) of Champneys Radiance Boosting Foamy Facial Wash or a similar product over the face and neck. Using a complexion brush (and ideally the Champneys Fresh Face Micro-Dermabrasion System brush) follow the following cleansing routine.

First, massage a facial cleanser onto your face. Using your hands or a brush sweep up your neck from the décolletage to the jaw line. Make small circles with the pads of your fingers along the chin to the ears and then back to the chin.

Circle, using the pads of the fingers of both hands, to cheeks and temples. With the pads of your fingers, press from the centre of the brow out to the temples – three times. With pads of fingers, press your upper lip from centre to outer corner and back again, three times.

Circle around your nostrils with the middle fingers. With the middle fingers, sweep from the side of the nostrils upwards and over the brows. Press into the temples with your finger pads. Hold and release.

Rinse off the cleanser.

Tone and exfoliate

Using one or two cotton wool pads, lightly sponge a toner (such as Champneys Skin Conditioning Gentle Toner) over your whole face and neck. Blot dry with a tissue.

Next, apply a gentle facial exfoliater such as Champneys Micro-Dermabrasion Facial Polish over the face and décolletage. Then, with a damp complexion sponge, repeat the face cleanse routine two times.

Rinse off the exfoliater and use the toner again.

Finish…

Apply a small amount of eye gel or cream. Moisturise your face and neck using your usual moisturiser.

To look your absolute bare-faced best, apply Champneys Perfect Skin Illuminating Beauty Balm and Moisture Miracle Rescue Balm to your lips – or use other products that give a tightening and brightening effect.

Harnessing the power of the sea

One of the reasons people return from a beach holiday feeling so fabulous is the effect of the sea air coupled with sea bathing. Negative ions are created by crashing water – waves, waterfalls, even the shower – and they have a powerfully energising effect. You can buy ionising units which can produce negative ions in your home, but nothing beats the vim of the 'real thing'.

You can bring the energising power of the sea into your life in other ways. Thalassotherapy is a term for the healing treatments that harness the power of the sea – seaweed, sea mud, sand and sea water. It improves skin conditions, relieves the pain which comes from arthritis and other forms of joint pain, stimulates the lymphatic system (thus boosting immunity), eases muscle pain and aids poor digestion. See page 65 for more about the lymphatic system.

At Champneys, our thalassotherapy pool sessions are amongst the most popular treatments. It's hard to duplicate the effect at home but you can still use the principles of thalassotherapy at home in an overnight invigorating programme.

Choose an evening when you can get to bed reasonably early and enjoy an Epsom salt bath – deeply relaxing, deeply detoxifying. Add around 500g of Epsom salts (from a chemist) to a warm bath. Light a candle and relax for about twenty minutes, sipping water continuously. Then wrap yourself up in a towel, change into cosy nightwear and bed socks and get into bed. (Don't shower off the salt.) Go straight to bed, and your sleep should be deep and dreamless. (Epsom salt baths are not recommended if you have high blood pressure or heart problems.)

Next morning, try Champneys Aqua Therapy Refining Salt Scrub – inspired by the thalassotherapy pools – to stimulate your skin prior to bathing. Alternatively, a handful of sea salt will work well to exfoliate your skin. Then rinse off with tepid water. Finish with a blast of cool water along the length of your spine. Try to stay under it for a count of twenty, then switch to tepid water again. Towel yourself dry, and moisturise. This is an ancient hydrotherapy technique for stimulating your nervous system and the good effects last for hours.

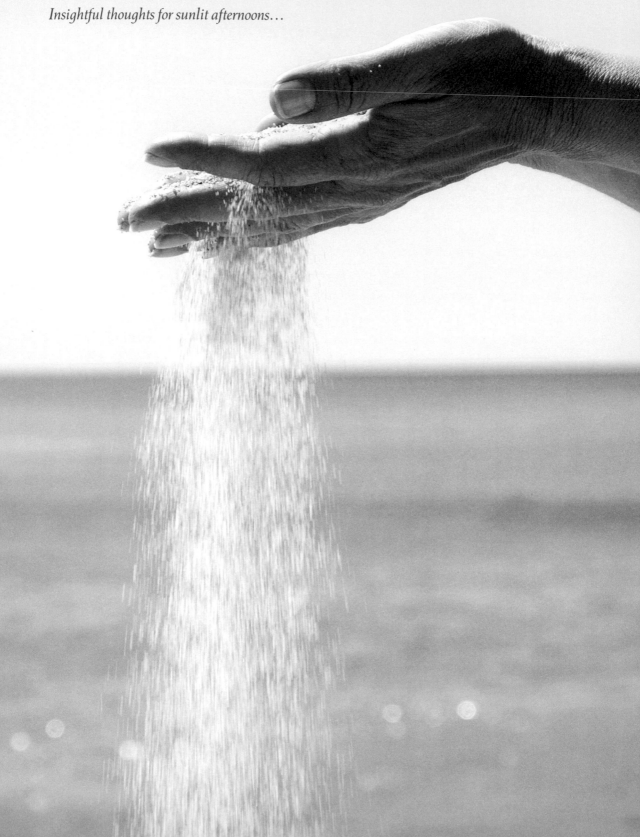

Insightful thoughts for sunlit afternoons…

Well-being

Reconnect with your passion

Sometimes it's hard to remember whose life you're living. There are so many demands on it from other people – people you are dependent on one way or another or whom you love so much that you don't begrudge the cost to you of meeting their demands.

Over the months, over the years we all lose sight of what we would really like to be doing if our time was our own. The result of that neglect over time is to rub away a little of our lustre. So try this:

• Sit quietly and remember as much as you can about yourself when you were around the age of twenty-one. What did you love to do? What did you love to spend time on? Who did you love to spend time with? Why? What did you long to be doing with your life? Write down as much as you can remember.

• Now go further back to when you were around sixteen or seventeen. Answer the questions. Get a clear idea of who you were in your mid-teens. Now go further back, say, to when you were eight. What did you love to do on school holidays? What did you love to do at school? Were there subjects you were good at but that you were never able to pursue? Again, write it down.

• Now look through what you've written, choose three activities that will allow you to express the person you used to be and then schedule time to spend on them in the next week or so. Carry on doing this on a weekly basis until your life begins to feel like your own again.

We don't change much in our intense interests and pleasures over the years. Reconnecting with what we love reminds us who we are and gives us energy. Our lives become richer and happier.

Be irresistible

The secret to magnetism is simple – love yourself. But remember that possessing the kind of high self-esteem that shines out isn't a constant, it's a work in progress.

Imagine if life just got easier, if everything you wanted seemed to flow towards you effortlessly. That's what the father of life coaching Thomas Leonard christened 'irresistible attraction'. Which is a fabulous way of saying 'sky-high self-esteem'. Your self-esteem is not a constant – it fluctuates depending on what is going on in your life. That is hugely comforting. Self-esteem levels can change. If your self-esteem levels are low, keeping an eye on them (by taking this quiz) and boosting them whenever you perceive a dip will make a big difference to how you experience life.

Answer 'yes' or 'no' to these statements based on how you're feeling right now, today.

	Yes	No
1. Does life seem unnecessarily complicated?	☐	☐
2. Do all your attempts to make life better seem to fail?	☐	☐
3. Do you feel you're at the mercy of your family, job or other people?	☐	☐
4. Are you feeling slightly sick at the thought of all you have to achieve by the end of the week?	☐	☐
5. Do you feel that, if you want something, you can make it happen?	☐	☐
6. Do you feel that you are expressing who you really are through your image, home, work or interests?	☐	☐

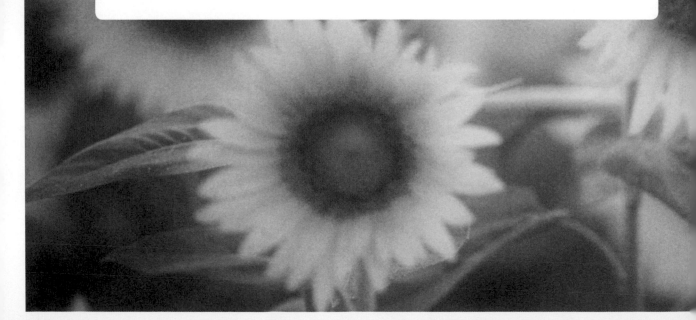

Answer 'no' to the first four questions and 'yes' to questions 5 and 6, and your self-esteem is high – for now. 'Yes' to the first four questions, 'no' to questions 5 or 6, and your self-esteem could use some work. Try these exercises.

• One characteristic of people with low self-esteem is that, deep down, they don't think they have much impact on their world. Those with healthy self-esteem know they make a difference. Easiest way of doing it? Pay a genuine compliment. Make someone else feel great about themselves. You remember a heartfelt compliment for the rest of your life, so be one of those memorable people.

• Set aside half an hour and write down every single thing you've been successful at or that you've completed successfully. Small things. Big things. When you run out of steam, look over the list and write down the qualities you needed to achieve each success – perseverance, courage, quick wit. Return to this list until you have at least 100 successes.

• Write down fifty words you would like to apply to yourself: for example, joyful, optimistic, strong, intuitive, confident. Pick a couple of these words that particularly appeal and try to act 'as if' you were this person already. This is incredibly powerful and the basis of the behavioural therapy NLP. Act like the person you want to be, copy their behaviour. One day you'll find you're not acting.

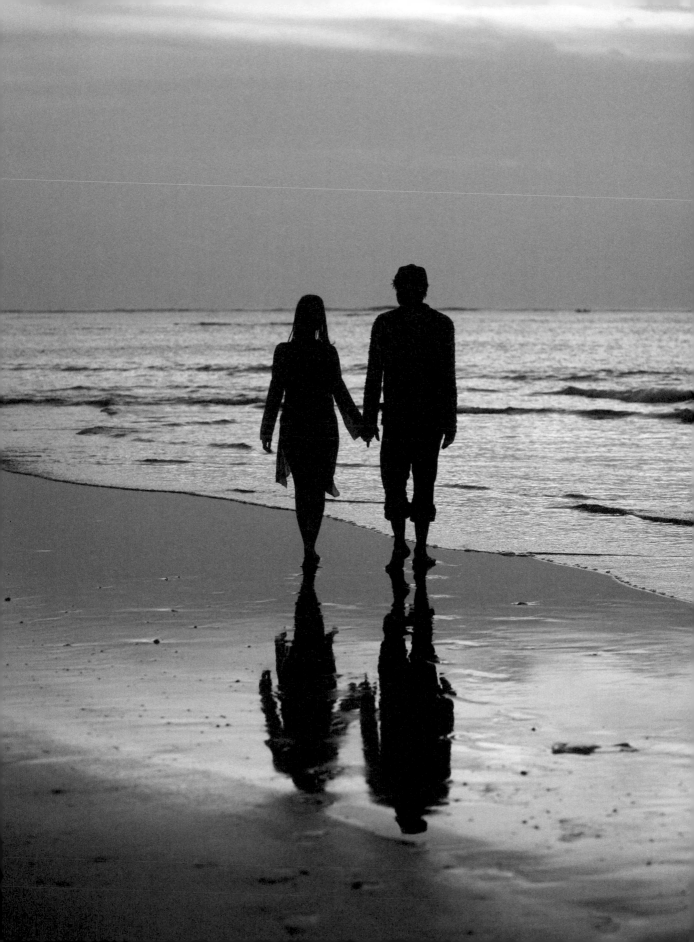

Creating 'perfect moments'

In the last few years neuroscientists, in their search to discover how we best can ensure happiness, have moved their attention from what's going wrong in the brains of depressed people to exploring what's going right in the brains of happy people. It seems to be quite simple. Happy people don't get so busy stressing about building a 'perfect' tomorrow that they forget to enjoy this 'perfect' day.

It turns out the surest, indeed the only, predictor of how happy you are going to be in the future is how good you are at being happy today. You can plan the perfect wedding, perfect party, perfect marriage, perfect career. But you have absolutely no idea if, when you get 'there', a perfect anything is going to be delivered. The only thing you can do is guarantee that today at least you will have a perfect moment – a moment where you pursue happiness and joy and feel inspired and contented. You may not be able to manage it for a whole day – but all of us, most of the time, can manage a minute or so.

Every day, plan to have a moment that reminds you that life is meant to be enjoyed. It might be first thing in the morning – a perfect cup of tea and a last snuggle in bed before you get up to face the day. It might be snatched late at night, listening to music by candlelight while the family sleeps. It could be sipping a glass of chilled wine as you sit in a deckchair while the sun slips behind your neighbour's roof. It could be during your yoga class, as you concentrate on the pull in your toned muscles, or while you smooth fragrant body lotion into your glowing skin after a rose-scented bath.

We all know the feeling that life is 'bigger' than ourselves and the sense of peace that comes with it. All you have to do is give yourself the space to feel it more often – ideally, once a day.

Planning for your perfect moment means that it is more likely to happen. And at the end of each day you will be able to say 'today, there were five minutes when I really enjoyed life'.

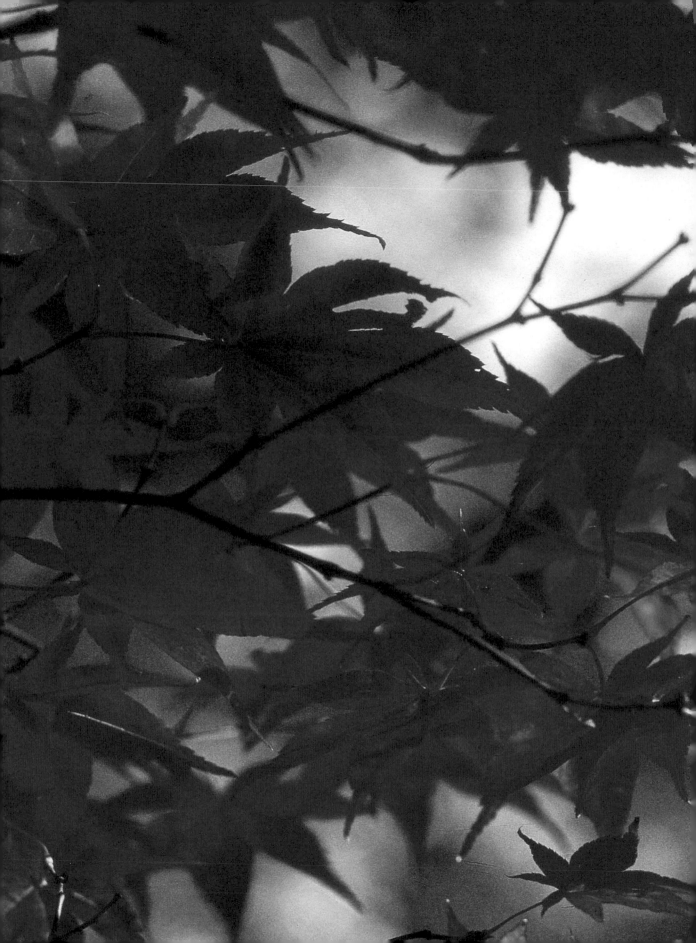

Autumn

Five ways to celebrate autumn

- Splash in some puddles and kick up piles of leaves. This gives you a great excuse to buy some gorgeous new wellies.

- Dress up for Halloween. Throw a party or go 'trick or treating' with the kids. Dunk for apples, carve pumpkins and tell ghost stories. The origins of Hallowe'en – celebrated by cultures around the world – lie in the ritual of remembering loved ones who have passed away. This October take time out to 'honour the ancestors', as they say in China, and appreciate their lasting gifts to you in whatever ritual feels appropriate.

- Make a perfect apple pie. Light a fire and indulge in all your domestic goddess fantasies. This is the time for relishing home comforts.

- Sprinkle cinnamon on your morning latte. It's been shown to help balance blood-sugar levels.

- Try adding a few drops of black pepper aromatherapy oil to your bath. Warming and comforting, it's perfect for soothing tired muscles. Autumn is the time to slow down. When your day allows, retreat to a quiet spot with a cosy blanket and take a quick nap. Closing your eyes for just twenty minutes makes you smarter, more productive and is also proven to reduce the chances of heart disease. It's also a great aid to productivity and creativity – Einstein, Brahms and Edison all thrived on an afternoon nap.

The harvest is home, you feel secure and safe

September is a great month to… enjoy the thrill of 'back to school' season. What about signing up for that evening class or course that's always interested you, becoming a member of your local theatre or concert hall, or simply treating yourself to a beautiful new notebook and pen so you can start keeping a journal.

October is a great month to… treasure your breasts (it's Breast Awareness month in the UK). Buy some beautiful new lingerie and treat yourself to a facial that extends to your décolletage. Have a mammogram if you've been invited for one; if not, check that you know exactly what your breasts should look and feel like. Resolve to keep an eye on any changes.

November is a great month to… throw a Thanksgiving dinner. All the guests have to share what they are most grateful for in the last year. Or invite only the people you have most cause to be grateful to in the last year and be sure they know how much you appreciate them. Grateful people are healthier people.

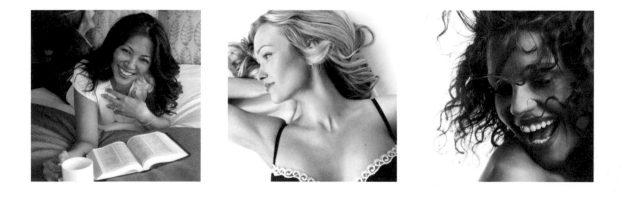

September... October... November... Autumn

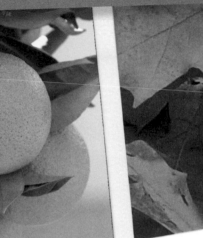

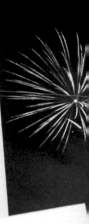

Power... autumn is the time to build up your body's strength with energising tonics and powerful Pilates.

Protect... your health, your back and your sanity against all the drains on your time and energy.

Unwind... with long walks in the country, kicking up golden leaves and enjoying long sessions in the bathroom, relaxing with rose-scented oils and unguents that will soothe your mind, heal your spirit and nurture your body.

Defend... your immune system with delicious meals, and your skin with seriously soothing treatments.

Balance... is restored in mind, body and spirit.

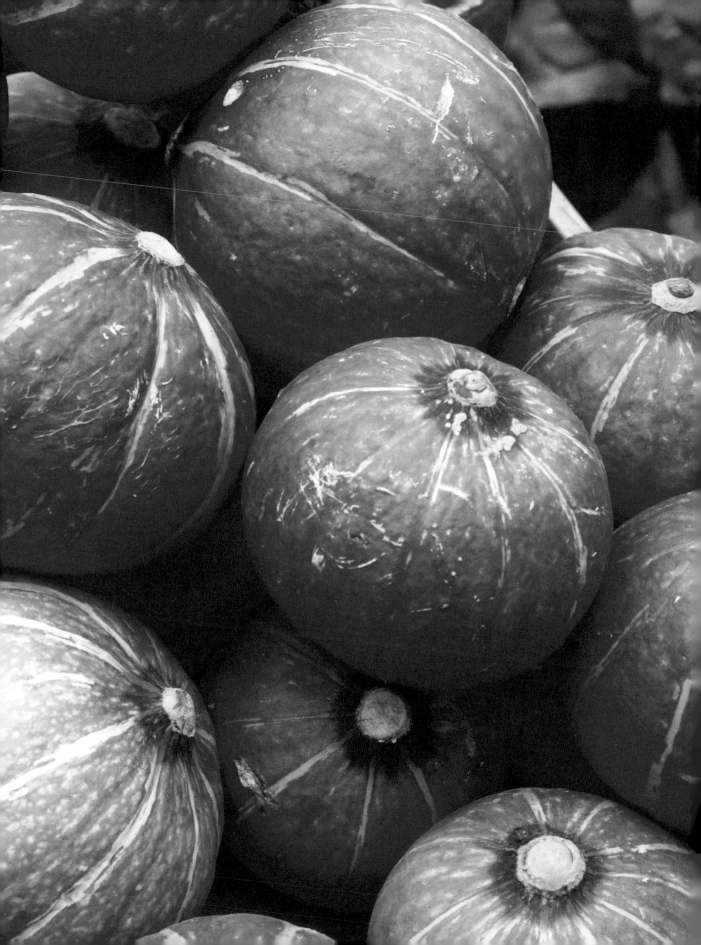

Eat

Enlivened by brisk winds, cool mornings and drifting leaves, autumn has its own invigorating energy after the sleepiness of summer. It's the perfect time to harness that energy and focus on how you can achieve a better balance in your life, thus protecting yourself from mental and physical stress. One of the most effective ways of doing that is via your diet.

The trouble with those well-worn words 'a well-balanced diet' is that most of us think we have one, when research proves that we don't. Government figures show that a large proportion of UK women are short of even some of the most basic nutrients found in many foods, such as calcium, iron and magnesium. The chance is high that such women are low in other nutrients necessary for optimal health.

Our ancestors ate seasonally and couldn't afford to be fussy, so they were exposed to a wider choice of foods. We, on the other hand, can choose to eat the same foods day in, day out which can lead to deficiencies. Not just that, but there is evidence that our food is just not as good as it used to be due to overprocessing, depleted soil, prolonged food storage and poor cooking techniques. For example:

• Vitamin C (required for healthy function by every cell in the body): we consume an estimated 90% less than our Stone Age predecessors.

 • Selenium (key for a healthy immune system): down by 50% in the last fifty years.

 • Silicon (essential for healthy hair, skin, nails): down 50% in the last hundred years.

 • Omega 3 fatty acids (play a crucial part in many key biochemical processes and are critical for healthy membrane function in all of our cells): intake estimated to be down 75% since Stone Age times.

We are not living the life we were developed for. Once, if we wanted to have food, we had to physically work to get it. It is perfectly possible to be overweight but undernourished; indeed, experts suggest that this 'type B' malnutrition is common in the West, and are predicting an epidemic of it.

The effect of vitamin and mineral depletion on overall health is catastrophic but not immediate. Slowly, subtly, things go wrong. By our sixties, five out of six of us have one or more of these chronic degenerative diseases: heart disease, diabetes, arthritis, cancer or osteoporosis. This reflects a lifetime of unhealthy lifestyle and poor nutrition. Micronutrient depletion can affect your immune system more quickly: you get cold after cold, feel run down and are at the mercy of every bug going.

The good news is that there is much you can do to boost your immunity – and improving your diet is central. With a little forethought you can supercharge your health and improve your chances of sailing through winter illness-free.

What is the immune system?

Your immune system is a complex multi-layered defence mechanism. Millions of look-out cells patrol your body in the bloodstream, returning to your heart via the lymphatic system. If these cells identify invading bugs, they 'neutralise' them and transport them to the lymph glands, located in the armpits, groin and under the jawline. When the immune system is fighting an invader, immune cells in the lymph glands multiply and the glands swell. Antibodies are produced, specifically designed for a particular target, and other immune cells may be mobilised to see off the invaders.

The ability of these cells to deal with invading bugs is determined by various factors. Genetics is one that you can't do much about. On the other hand, your nutritional state and psychological and emotional health affect your immune system, and both are under your control.

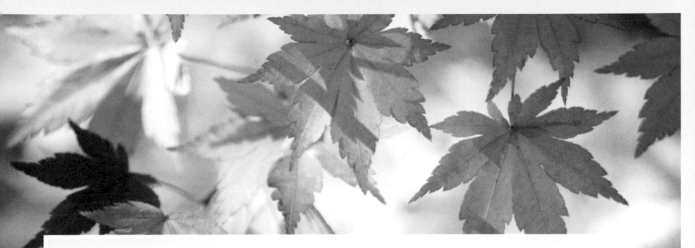

Are you in good shape?

Try this quiz to find out if your immune system is in good shape.

	Yes	No
1. Have you had an ear infection in the last year?	☐	☐
2. Do you often get ill when on holiday, or just after you return?	☐	☐
3. Do you suffer from sore throats more than twice a year?	☐	☐
4. Do you smoke?	☐	☐
5. Do you suffer from hay fever?	☐	☐
6. Do you suffer from eczema or dermatitis?	☐	☐
7. Do you usually get more than two colds a year?	☐	☐
8. Do you take a multivitamin/mineral supplement every day?	☐	☐
9. If you nick your finger with a knife, is it usually well on the way to healing by the next day?	☐	☐

Score one point for every 'yes' except for the last two questions, where you score one point for a 'no'. Any score of three or more indicates that your immune system could do with a boost. Question 7, in particular, is telling. Suffering from more than two colds a year is a good indication that your immune system needs a boost.

It's time to take a tonic or two

At this time of year, it's traditional to start taking a tonic to boost your immune system. Choose from these.

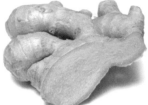

- Ginger. Swap one of your usual cups of tea for ginger tea instead. Boil a chopped root of ginger for 10–15 minutes and drink the liquid. Or add chopped ginger root to juice or soup.

- Siberian ginseng. It can boost aspects of your immune system, as well as blocking the immune dampening effects of the stress hormones. Try taking 2–4 ml of tincture three times a day or a 150mg capsule of standardised ginseng root. It's best to take a two-week break from consumption every two months.

- Echinacea. There is some good scientific evidence that Echinacea works despite some reports in the press that it doesn't, and people who take it consistently are often evangelical about its ability to reduce the number of colds they get. Choose a good quality supplement of Echinacea purpurea. Like ginseng, it's best to take a two-week break every two months.

Ailsa Higgins, Champneys' nutritionist, recommends taking a combination of Siberian ginseng and Echinacea at the very first sign of a cold or flu.

Supplementary benefit

You should also think about taking a multivitamin and mineral supplement. A research study published in *The Lancet* found that people taking a supplement had had fewer infections, were generally healthier, and their blood tests showed evidence of a stronger immune system.

You can cut down on sick days. Eating to boost immunity means tweaking your usual healthy diet:

• Protein is essential for the rapid production of immune cells, so when you're exposed to an infection, ensure you eat enough protein. Not too much though: protein uses up vitamin B6 in its processing, which is a key immune system nutrient. Aim for two palm-sized portions daily.

• Essential fats (from nuts, seeds and fish) boost immunity.

• Lots of fruit and vegetables: they're packed with the vitamins and minerals needed to fight infection.

Especially useful are sweet potato, squash, carrot, broccoli, tomatoes, watercress, beetroot and berries. Shitake mushrooms and pears both contain special polysaccharides like those present in Echinacea which can boost the immune system.

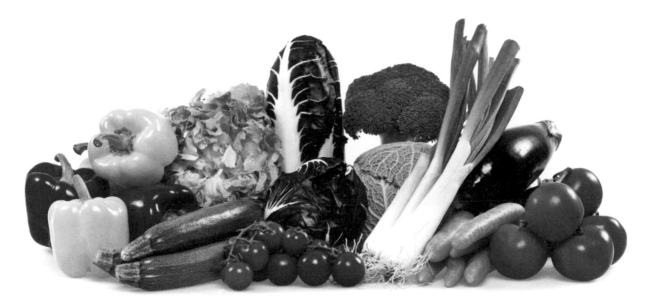

Your autumn weekly prescription

Making subtle changes to your diet can make a real difference to how well you are going to stay over the next few months. Make a concentrated effort to increase intake of these foods from September onwards – and by the time the 'cold season' hits, you should be armoured against it with a tip-top immune system.

Oily fish such as salmon, mackerel, herring

These are rich in omega-3 fats which protect the lungs from colds and respiratory infections by reducing inflammation and increasing airflow.
Weekly prescription: two or three times a week.

Liver, kidney, fish and shellfish.

These are rich in selenium which boosts cellular immunity. Weekly prescription: once or twice a week.

Oats and barley

These are loaded with beta-glucans. Scientists have recently recognised the value of this fibre; Norwegian research discovered that it is more potent than Echinacea in boosting antioxidant capacity. In animal studies, beta-glucans cut the risk of infection from a whole slew of viruses including flu. In human studies, it boosts immunity and speeds up wound healing.
Weekly prescription: seven times a week at least. Porridge for breakfast makes this easy!

Natural live yoghurt

The 'friendly' bacteria found in yoghurt protect the gut. It's been discovered that a healthy supply of these reduces the risk of colds and flu viruses by 'dealing' with them before they get a chance to take hold in the body. A Swedish study revealed that taking probiotics reduced sick days by one third.
Weekly prescription: seven times a week – one serving a day, equivalant to a small pot.

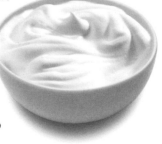

Chicken soup

Chicken soup is a superlative immunity-boosting food. Chicken is rich in the amino acid cysteine (which has a similar structure to bronchial drugs) and the vegetables supply antioxidants. US research has shown that shop-bought chicken soup does the job by keeping white cells circulating freely round the body, which results in a lessening of symptoms. But home-made chicken soup is worth making because you can add extra garlic and onions, rich in allicin and quercetin respectively, which will help thin mucus and increase the soup's immune-boosting power.

Weekly prescription: once a week (and more if you feel that you might be going down with something).

Tea

Swapping a few of your regular brews of coffee for tea will help boost your virus-fighting levels of interferon by a factor of ten in just two weeks. This is due to tea's high level of L-theanine which is found in green and black tea, and in decaff versions, too. And dunking your tea bag vigorously gives you five times more antioxidants.

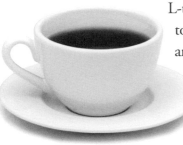

Weekly prescription: three to four times a day.

Dairy and wheat foods tend to increase mucus production. So cut down on these to help a stuffed nose if you feel a cold coming on.

The garlic dilemma

Garlic is a great cold fighter, thanks largely to its active ingredient, allicin. British researchers gave 146 people either a placebo or a garlic extract for twelve weeks: the garlic takers were two-thirds less likely to catch a cold. Garlic is a natural antibacterial, antiviral, antibiotic, antihistamine, anticoagulant and expectorant. (It lowers cholesterol and blood pressure, lowers blood-sugar levels too, and reduces your risk of colon cancer and stomach cancer by between 30–50%.)

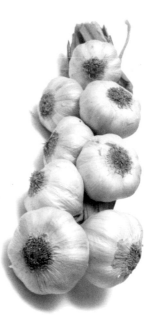

For a therapeutic dose, you should eat around one to two crushed cloves a day. A good way of getting enough garlic is to put some mashed-up garlic in a juicer first thing in the morning and swallow it down quickly! Keep a pot of parsley on your kitchen window and chew a mouthful afterwards. It is a natural breath cleanser and neutralises the garlic smell. Alternatively you could take a garlic supplement.

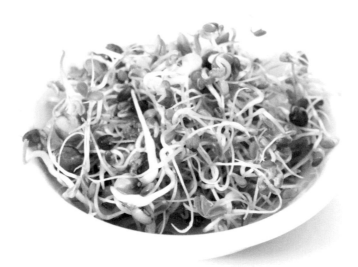

'Sprouted seeds are packed with vitamins and enzymes. They're cheap, quick and easy to grow on a small space on a kitchen shelf, and produce handfuls of the freshest food you'll ever eat!'

– AILSA HIGGINS, CHAMPNEYS' NUTRITIONIST

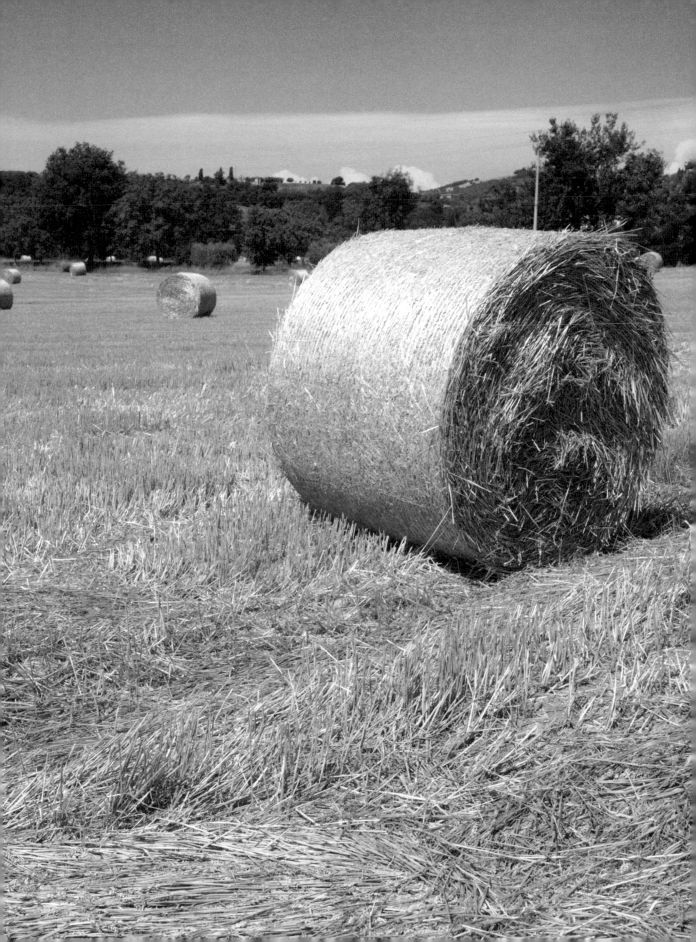

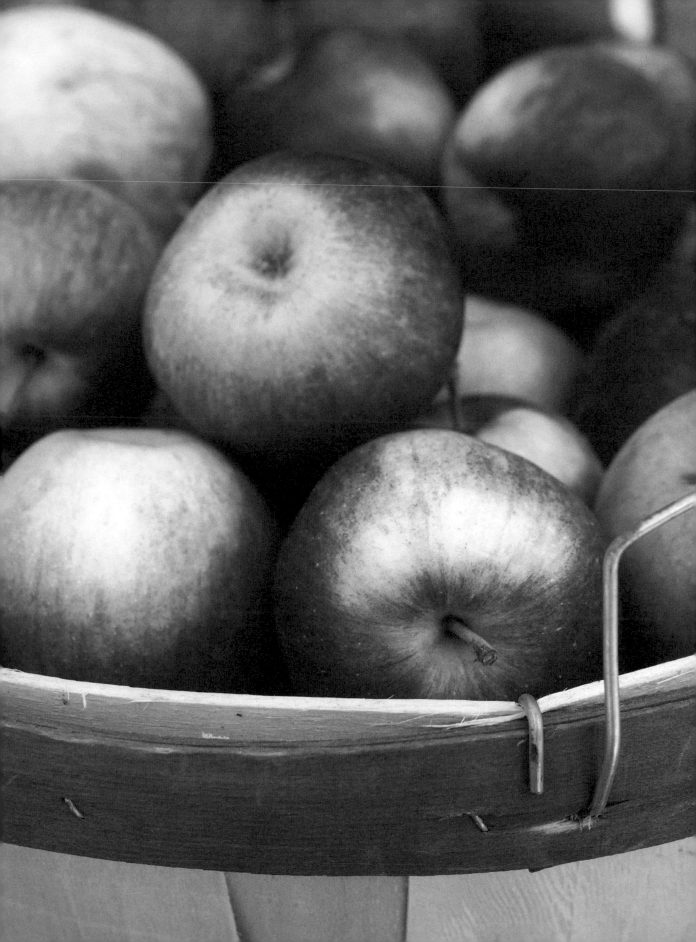

Inspiration to eat well...

Breakfasts

Energy smoothie
(serves 1)
1 large ripe banana, peeled and sliced
200ml semi-skimmed milk
1 tbsp smooth nut butter
A pinch of ground nutmeg and cinnamon
A handful of ice cubes

Place all the ingredients in a blender and whizz until smooth. Then add the ice cubes and whizz again, until the cubes have been well broken up. Pour into a tall glass and serve immediately

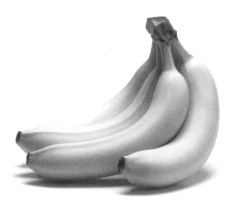

This is a great energy boost after exercise. Bananas are an excellent source of potassium which helps keep blood-pressure levels healthy. Nuts provide healthy fats, to support healthy skin and joints, the nervous system and immune system. Nuts are also packed with important vitamins and minerals such as vitamin E, B vitamins and magnesium. These nutrients help with exercise recovery, metabolism and energy production.

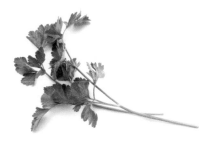

Poached finnan haddock

(serves 1)

½ a plum tomato

A little olive oil

About 200ml milk and water

175g natural-smoked haddock fillet

Sprig of flat leaf parsley, to serve

Lemon wedge, to serve

Season the plum tomato, brush with a little oil and put it under a grill. While it is cooking, bring a saucepan containing just enough milk and water to cover the haddock fillet to the simmer and then place the fish in it. Gently poach it for 3–4 minutes, depending on the thickness of the fillet. When it is done, lift the haddock out of the poaching liquor, drain it and put it onto a plate with the grilled plum tomato. Garnish with the flat leaf parsley and lemon wedge and serve immediately.

Autumnal apple, pear and blackberry juice

(serves 1)

3 apples, chopped but not peeled

2 firm and ripe pears, chopped but not peeled

A punnet of fresh blackberries

Soya or natural yoghurt, to taste

Blend the fruit, and strain if required to remove any seeds. For a complete breakfast, blend in some soya or live natural yoghurt.

If you leave the skin on the apples and pears, you maximise fibre and nutrient content.

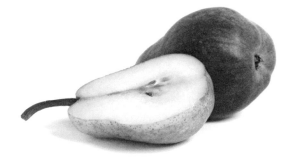

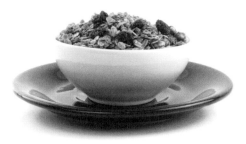

Champneys' granola

(makes about a kilo; store in an airtight
container for up to a month)

2 tbsp rapeseed oil

125ml agave or maple syrup

2 tbsp wild flower honey

1 tsp vanilla extract

300g rolled oats

100g sunflower and pumpkin seeds, mixed

4 tbsp sesame seeds

100g chopped nuts

50g wheatgerm

50g desiccated coconut

60g dried chopped dates

60g dried chopped apricots

75g raisins

Zest of one orange

Zest of one lemon

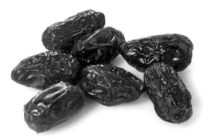

Pre-heat the oven to 150ºC / gas mark 2. Mix together the oil, maple syrup, honey and vanilla extract in a large bowl. Tip in all the other ingredients except the coconut, dried fruit and zests, and mix them well.

Now tip the granola onto a large baking sheet and spread it out evenly. Bake it for 15 minutes, then mix in the coconut, dried fruit and zests and bake for another 15 minutes.

Remove it from the oven and scrape onto a flat tray to cool. Serve with cold milk or yoghurt for breakfast, or as a snack.

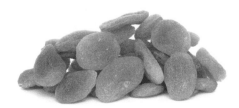

Lunches and main courses

Sweet potato soup
(serves 2)
1 onion, diced
1 tsp garlic puree
1 leek, chopped
1 sweet potato, peeled and diced
Salt and pepper
600ml vegetable stock
1 tsp fresh chopped parsley, to garnish

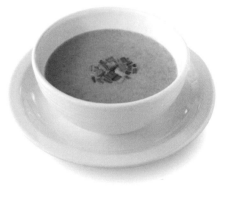

Using a saucepan, sweat the onions and garlic in a little olive oil. Add the leek and sweet potato, season with salt and pepper and sauté for five minutes. Add the vegetable stock, bring to the boil then reduce the heat and simmer for 15–20 minutes. Blend until smooth. Then serve, garnished with chopped parsley.

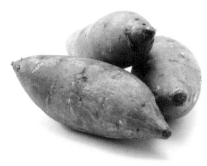

Why this is the perfect immunity-boosting soup
Orange-fleshed sweet potatoes are a great source of the antioxident beta-carotene, important for the skin, eyes and lungs. This, together with its vitamin C, helps support the immune system and prevent premature ageing. It also has a type of soluble fibre that is gentle and supportive of the digestive system, and which may also be helpful in lowering cholesterol levels. Garlic has antibacterial properties and supports the growth of the friendly 'probiotic' bacteria that line the digestive tract and protect us from colds. Onions are good source of quercetin, a natural anti-inflammatory.

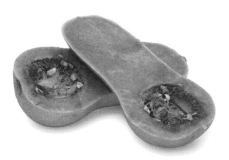

Mrs Murphy's butternut squash soup

(serves 4–6)
1 whole butternut squash, peeled and diced
5 medium carrots, peeled and diced
A little olive oil
6 plum tomatoes, chopped
A small bunch of basil, chopped
A small bunch of tarragon, chopped
1.2 litres vegetable stock
Salt

Place the butternut squash and carrots in a saucepan with the olive oil and sweat them until they are soft, but don't let them start to catch – give them a good stir. Add the tomatoes and herbs and continue cooking, still stirring, until the tomatoes are softening. Add the vegetable stock and season with a little salt; bring the pan up to a simmer and cook the soup for 20–30 minutes. When the vegetables are soft, remove the pan from the heat and blend the soup with a hand blender until it is smooth (you could, of course, use an ordinary blender). Pass the soup through a sieve, pressing all the liquid from the pulp. Check the soup for seasoning and serve immediately.

Beetroot and orange salad

(serves 1)
2 medium cooked beetroot, diced
2 oranges, peeled and cut into segments
1 shallot, finely diced
¼ tbsp fresh tarragon

For the dressing:
60ml natural yoghurt
Grated zest of half an orange
½ tsp wholegrain mustard
Salt and pepper

First, make the dressing. Put the yoghurt, orange zest and mustard in a bowl and mix them together well. Check for seasoning and add salt and pepper if necessary. Mix all the salad ingredients, add the dressing and toss everything together. Serve immediately.

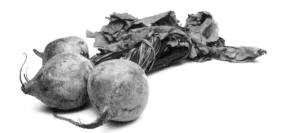

Mushroom and goat's cheese melt with pesto

(serves 2)

4 large flat mushrooms

Salt and pepper

A little olive oil

1 beef tomato

150g goat's cheese

For the pesto:

A handful of rocket

1 garlic clove

25g pine nuts

25g Parmesan cheese

100ml olive oil

Mixed salad leaves, to serve

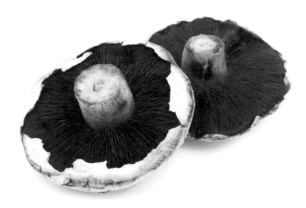

Pre-heat the oven to 150ºC / gas mark 2. Peel the mushrooms, season them with salt and pepper and drizzle with a little olive oil. Put them on a tray and cook in the oven for 10–15 minutes. While they are cooking, put all the ingredients for the pesto into a food processor and whizz, adding the oil last. When the mushrooms are cooked, remove them from the oven. Layer the tomato and goat's cheese on top of the mushrooms with the goat's cheese on the top. Place them under a hot grill to melt the cheese a little.

To serve, put on a plate with the mixed salad leaves and drizzle some pesto around them.

Goats' cheese is a source of selenium, a powerful antioxidant.

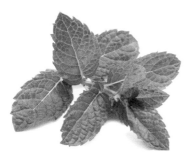

Roast lamb rump steaks with Moroccan couscous and mint yoghurt

(serves 4)

150ml vegetable stock

75g couscous

1 tbsp of olive oil

½ tsp cumin powder

½ tsp coriander powder

½ tsp mixed spice powder

50g mixed peppers, diced

5 dried apricots, diced

25g sultanas

1 slice of onion, finely chopped

A garlic clove, roasted

A large sprig of mint, chopped

A sprig of coriander, chopped

4 x 175g lamb rump steaks

100ml natural yoghurt

Salt and pepper

Heat the vegetable stock. Place the couscous in a large bowl and add the stock; stir until all the stock has been soaked up by the couscous and leave it for 3 minutes. Then add the olive oil and stir again. Leave it to cool down slightly. When cool, add the spices, mixed pepper, diced apricots and sultanas and mix everything together. Then add the onion, the garlic clove, half the chopped mint and all the chopped coriander, mix again and set aside.

Pre-heat the oven to 180ºC / gas mark 4. Put a frying pan on a high heat and add the lamb steaks. You just want to seal in the juices, so only cook them very briefly. When they have been sealed on both sides, transfer them to a roasting tin and put the tin in the oven. How long you cook them for will depend on how you like your lamb. They will be rare after 15 minutes, medium after 20 minutes and well done after 25–30 minutes. When the lamb is cooked as you like it, remove it from the oven and let it rest, covered, for 5 minutes.

Now prepare the yoghurt dressing by adding the rest of the chopped mint to the natural yoghurt. Add salt and pepper to taste. Cover the couscous bowl with cling film, pierce a few holes in the film and reheat it in the microwave for 1 minute. Serve the lamb steaks on a bed of couscous accompanied by the mint yoghurt.

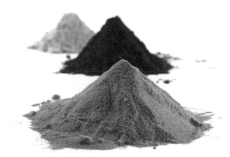

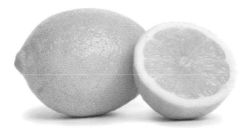

Courgette and lemon pilaff

(serves 4–6)

450g Basmati rice

2 tbsp olive or cold-pressed rapeseed oil

2 onions, peeled and chopped

4 garlic cloves, crushed

6 medium courgettes, chopped

2 unwaxed lemons, cut into quarters and pips removed

1.2 litres vegetable stock

A handful of chopped coriander, to serve

Rinse the rice under running cold water. Heat the olive oil and gently cook the onion and garlic until transparent. Stir in the rice, courgettes and lemon and cook for a few minutes. Pour in the stock, bring to the boil, cover and cook on a low heat for about 15 minutes until all the stock is absorbed and the rice is tender. Season the pilaff and stir in the chopped coriander; serve immediately.

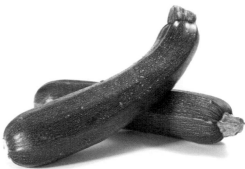

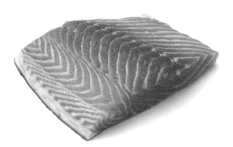

Salmon and herb fishcakes

(serves 4)

500g salmon

500g floury potatoes (such as King Edwards)

A small knob of butter

Salt and pepper

1 tbsp finely chopped parsley

Zest of 1 lemon

1 egg, beaten

100g fresh breadcrumbs

A little olive or rapeseed oil

Mixed leaf salad, to serve

Lemon wedges, to serve

Pre-heat the oven to 190ºC / gas mark 5. Put the salmon in a baking dish with a little water in the bottom, and cover the dish with foil. Put it in the oven for about 15 minutes until cooked (the colour changes when it is done). Let it cool down, then remove the skin and flake the fish into a bowl.

Boil the potatoes until they are cooked and mash them with a small knob of butter and salt and pepper to season; stir in the chopped parsley and the zest of one of the lemons. Now fold in the salmon carefully and allow the mixture to cool right down.

Using your hands, make the mixture into eight cakes and then brush them on both sides with beaten egg. Place the breadcrumbs in a bowl and gently cover both sides of each fishcake with them. Put the fishcakes on a plate (not on top of one another) and chill them for an hour in the fridge.

Heat a little oil in a non-stick pan and cook the fishcakes in batches for 2–3 minutes on each side until golden brown, keeping them warm in a low oven as you work. Serve them with salad and wedges of lemon.

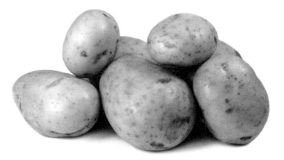

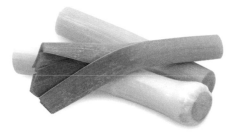

Oven-baked field mushrooms and leeks with herb crumb and red wine dressing

(serves 4)

4 field mushrooms, medium size

Salt and pepper

A little olive oil

1 medium onion, finely chopped

1 garlic clove

300ml vegetable stock

2 leeks, sliced

300ml low-fat cream

For the herb crumb:

1 tbsp butter

1 shallot

1 tbsp fresh, chopped, mixed herbs, such as flat leaf parsley, thyme, chervil and chives

4 slices of wholemeal bread, made into breadcrumbs

For the dressing:

1 egg

About ½ tbsp red wine vinegar

150ml walnut oil

150ml groundnut oil

About ½ tbsp Dijon mustard

Mixed leaves, to serve

Pre-heat the oven to 160ºC / gas mark 2.5. Peel the field mushrooms and remove the stalks, place them on a baking tray, then season with salt and pepper and drizzle with olive oil. Put them in the oven and bake for 10–15 minutes. Don't switch the oven off; you will need it again.

Now put the chopped onion and garlic into a pan with a little more olive oil and gently sweat them; don't allow them to colour. When they have softened, add the vegetable stock and bring to the boil. Once boiling, add the leeks. Bring it back to the boil and remove the pan from the heat. Put a colander over a clean bowl and strain the leeks, collecting the stock in the pan. Put that pan back on the heat and reduce the liquor by one third. Reduce the heat to very low, and add the low-fat cream; simmer gently for 5 minutes. Check the seasoning, remove from the heat and, when cool, mix with the leeks.

To make the crumb, warm the butter in a pan with chopped shallot. Put the breadcrumbs into a bowl, add the chopped herbs and a little salt and pepper. Add the shallot and butter to the crumb, and mix together.

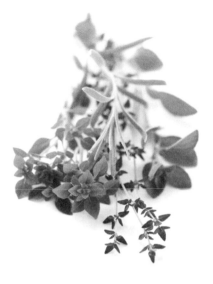

Prepare the dressing next. Place the egg, vinegar and Dijon mustard in a bowl, then gently whisk in the oils, and season.

To assemble, spoon the leeks into the centre of each mushroom and place the crumble mixture on top. Put them on a baking tray and bake in the oven for 10–15 minutes until they are golden brown. Arrange on top of some mixed seasonal leaves and drizzle the dressing around. Any left-over dressing can be kept in the fridge for up to a week.

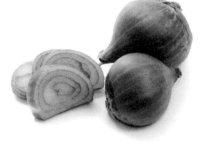

Puddings

Granny Smith jelly with cinnamon cream
(serves 4)
2 Granny Smith apples
Half a lemon
225ml sweet white wine
150ml apple juice
75ml orange juice
75g caster sugar
A clove
4 leaves of gelatine, soaked according to packaging instructions

To serve:
125g crème fraiche
20g icing sugar
A small pinch of cinnamon

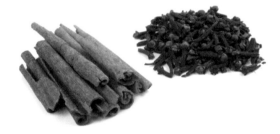

Make this jelly the day before you want to serve it, so that it is well set.

Core and grate the Granny Smith apples; put them straight into a bowl of water with a squeeze of lemon juice in it. Pour the wine, apple juice and orange juice into a saucepan, add another squeeze of lemon, the sugar and the clove and bring it to the boil. Drain the grated apple well and add it to the liquid. Simmer for a few minutes until the apple is soft. Now squeeze the water from the gelatine and stir the gelatine into the pan until it has dissolved. Remove the pan from the heat and leave it to cool.

Strain the jelly through a sieve into a jug, pressing on the apple in the sieve with the back of a spoon to extract all the flavour. Divide into serving glasses, or pour the jelly into a pudding bowl, and put it in the fridge to set overnight. Before serving, whisk the crème fraiche with the icing sugar and a pinch of cinnamon and spoon it onto the jellies.

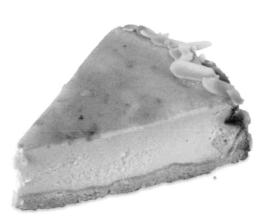

Baked American cheesecake
(serves 8–10)
1 x 25cm sponge disc
225g caster sugar
3 tbsp cornflour
750g low-fat soft cream cheese
2 eggs, beaten
1 tbsp vanilla essence
300ml whipping cream

Pre-heat the oven to 180ºC / gas mark 4.
Grease a 25cm cake tin and trim the sponge
disc to fit it perfectly; set it to one side. In
a large bowl, mix the sugar and cornflour
together, then beat in the cream cheese
and make sure they are all mixed together
thoroughly. Add the beaten eggs and vanilla
essence, and mix those in well too. Now add
the cream, stirring slowly but thoroughly,
to give a smooth mix. Pour this cheesecake
mixture on top of the sponge base in the cake
tin. Sit the cake tin in a roasting tin with a
small amount – not more than 3mm – of
water around it, and put it in the oven. Bake
it for 45–50 minutes or until it is golden and
set. Allow the cheesecake to cool in the tin
before serving.

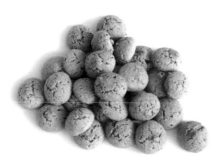

Caramelised Marsala pears with polenta and almond biscuits

(serves 4)

100ml Marsala wine

25g sugar

4 ripe pears, peeled and cut into quarters or sixths depending on their size

A pinch of ground mixed spice

100g blackberries

3 tbsp mascarpone cheese

100ml low-fat Greek yoghurt

Zest of 1 unwaxed lemon

For the biscuits:

50g olive oil spread

50g caster sugar

25g polenta

50g ground almonds

50g wholemeal flour

Make the biscuits first. Cream the olive oil spread and sugar together and add the polenta, the ground almonds and then the flour. Mix and leave to rest for 20 minutes, and pre-heat the oven to 180ºC / gas mark 4. Roll out the biscuit dough and cut it into 12 biscuits, using a 5cm plain round cutter. Put the circles of biscuit dough onto a non-stick baking tray and cook them in the oven for 15–20 minutes, until golden brown. Cool them on a wire rack.

Heat a large frying pan over a high heat, and add the Marsala and sugar. Stir briefly and, once the sugar has dissolved, reduce the heat. Once the sugar and Marsala have caramelised (watch for the change in colour), add the pears and cook until lightly coloured, taking care not to overcook the fruit. Strain the pears using a slotted spoon and put them to one side. Transfer the juices to a non-stick saucepan and boil to reduce by two-thirds. Then add the mixed spice and blackberries, cook for a further two minutes and leave to cool.

Mix the mascarpone, yoghurt and lemon zest, and assemble the dessert with layers of biscuits (3 per person), mascarpone mixture and the pears. Spoon the blackberries and juices around the edge of the plate and serve at once.

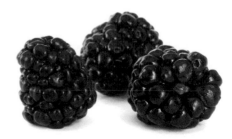

In autumn, choose these seasonal foods

Damsons, plums, apples, sweetcorn, figs, elderberries, parsnips, beetroot, chestnuts, partridge, oysters, grouse and autumn lamb.

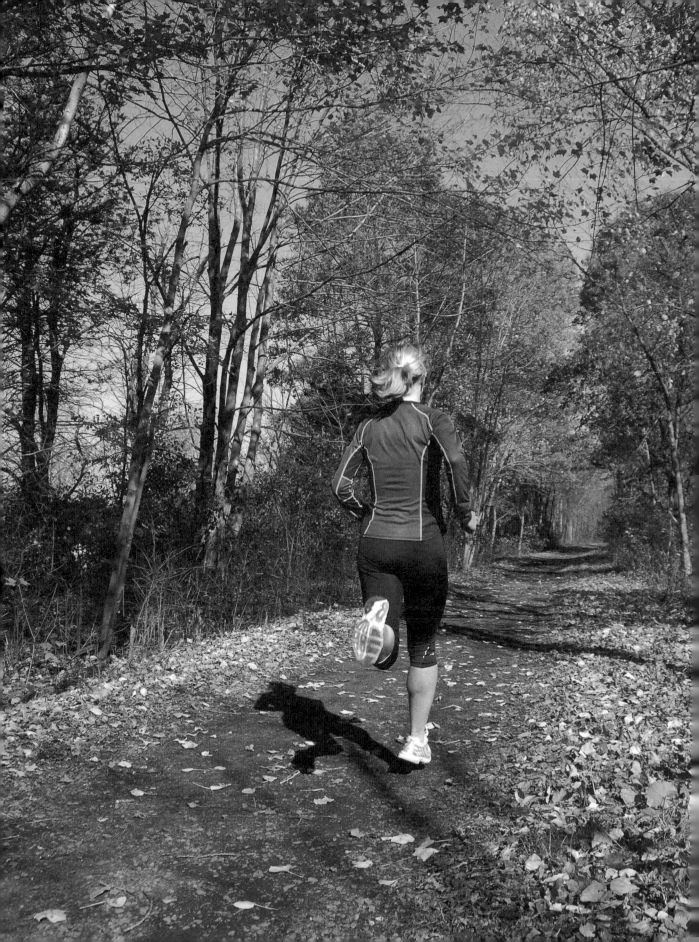

Move

The theme of autumn is building up strength, achieving balance and protecting yourself. Pilates is a superb exercise for achieving all of these goals. It builds core strength but is loved by its many devotees for the way it sculpts bodies and seems to elongate muscles. Doing regular Pilates means you walk taller and look slimmer. The Champneys' at-home programme, originally created by Alan Herdman, the UK's leading practitioner of the Pilates technique, is easy to follow and takes very little time. However, if you are new to Pilates, it is worth seeking out a local class to get the feel of the slow, controlled and precise movements that can have such a profound effect on the way you look and feel.

One of the important aspects of the Pilates technique is that it starts with fundamentals – posture and breathing – and all exercises build on these foundations. You should be familiar with how neutral spine (see page 114) feels and maintain it during these exercises even though you are on the floor. In addition, before beginning each exercise, draw your navel in towards your spine to help form a strong centre and safeguard your back.

Your goals are to concentrate on your alignment and posture above all, so do not rush any of the exercises, even if they feel easy. Maintain awareness of the whole body and don't let one part take over. Always check that the whole body is in the correct position, relaxed and lengthened, and focus on deep, slow, rhythmical breathing with effort performed on the out breath. You may find that slow classical music will help to keep your breathing steady. Please note that these suggestions assume that you are in good general health. If you are pregnant, or have any known health condition please consult your doctor and a qualified Pilates teacher.

Warm up – breathing

Lie on your back with your knees bent and feet hip-width apart. Make sure that you lie straight with no tension in your neck and shoulders. Support your head with a folded towel and place a rolled-up towel between your knees; this is not to squeeze but to keep the pelvis central throughout the exercise. Place your hands on your ribs, just below the arm pits. Breathe in through your nose and feel your ribs lift your hands upwards. Breathe out through your mouth and feel your ribs move in again. Try to create a slow, deep rhythm. This is how you need to breathe throughout the exercises. Repeat for ten slow, deep breaths.

Static abs

This is a continuation of the previous exercise which transforms the breathing into a movement and teaches the basis for many Pilates exercises. Lie on your back with your knees bent and feet hip-width apart. Place a folded towel between your knees and another under your head so that your neck and spine are straight. Relax your arms by your sides and let your shoulder sink into the floor. Breathe in, and as you breathe out draw your navel (abdomen) down towards your spine so that the abdominal muscles are scooped into a spoon shape. Release and repeat ten times.

Pelvic tilts

Lie on your back, with your knees bent, feet hip-width apart. Place a rolled-up towel between your knees and another towel under your head. Relax your upper body. Breathe in, and as you breathe out draw your navel down towards your spine and lift your pelvic floor muscles. (These are a hammock of muscles running from the pubic bone at the front to the anus at the back.)

As you lift your pelvic floor, tilt your pelvis so that you feel the hollow in your lower back flatten and then lift your pelvis a few centimetres off the floor. Think of your abdominals helping to curve the spine as you lift. Make sure you aren't squeezing your thighs together or creating tension in your upper body. The abdominal and pelvic floor muscles should be doing all the work. Breathe in and as you breathe out slowly roll your lower back and pelvis back down to the ground again. Repeat slowly ten times.

Caution: If you have lordosis – a pronounced arch in your lower back – try doing this exercise with your lower legs resting on a low chair. If you have kyphosis – a forward curve in the upper back – support your head and shoulders with cushions so that they feel comfortable and are not forced down into the floor as you exercise.

Buttock squeeze

Lie face down with a pillow to support your abdomen and a small cushion between your thighs. Rest your forehead on your hands on another folded towel. If this feels uncomfortable in your upper back, try slipping a small cushion under each shoulder. The upper body should be relaxed. Breathe in, and as you breathe out squeeze your buttocks towards each other. You should feel the abdominal muscles engage and your lower back gently lengthen. Don't let your legs turn inwards. Hold the squeeze for four seconds. Repeat ten times.

Heel lifts

It's very important that you raise your leg in a straight line for this exercise. Ask someone to watch you doing it and correct you if necessary. Or imagine a line that runs directly between your heel and your fingertips on each side, and don't waver from it.

Lie face down on the floor with a pillow under your abdomen. Rest your forehead and left hand on a folded towel. Extend your right arm out along the floor by your head. Stretch each leg a little to make sure they are straight and parallel. Breathe in. As you breathe out, very slowly bend your right leg until your knee is at a right angle. Imagine your right heel runs in a straight line towards your right fingers. Don't jerk, and keep your foot soft. You should be able to feel the muscles in the back of your thigh working. Breathe in to lower your right leg to the ground. Repeat 10 times with each leg.

Caution: If you find that your leg jerks or shakes while doing this exercise, try making the movement smaller. One way to do this is to place a cushion under your feet and lift from a raised position. Those with knee problems might find it helps if you place a folded towel under each thigh so that your knees aren't pushed into the floor. If you experience any discomfort, just stop.

The arrow

This exercise gives a great stretch to the upper back as you slide your shoulder blades down and lengthen your neck away from your body.

Lie on your front with your abdomen supported by a pillow and your forehead rested on a folded towel. Place a cushion under each shoulder if you find it helps you to relax your upper back. Rest your arms by your sides. Your legs should be hip-width apart and the heels turned slightly inward. Breathe in. As you breathe out, engage your abdominal muscles and lift the palms of your hands upward, to about the level of your bottom. Keep resting your head on the towel. Feel the stretch. Breathe in to return to the starting position. Repeat 10 times.

Variation: As you lift the palm of your hands upwards, try sliding your shoulder blades down your back and lifting your head and breastbone, stretching them forward. Keep your upper spine in a straight line and don't tilt your head back.

Louise Day, Champneys' Well-being Director, says:

'If you get out of the exercise habit, no matter how long you've been away, start small, even if it's a ten-minute walk after dinner or before work. It's a signal to yourself that you are recommitting. Stop kicking yourself. That "why bother" attitude can keep you stuck in a self-defeating cycle – so instead of feeding on that guilt, use it to propel you forward. Realise that slipping back into old habits doesn't mean you've failed – we all need to go back to old behaviours to test them out. Remember how it felt to be that sedentary person as opposed to the new, more active person you have started to become. Making exercise a habit is a journey, not a destination. The only difference between a person who fails at exercise and a person who succeeds comes down to never giving up. Even fitness professionals miss sessions – the difference is that they start again.'

Curl-ups

The Pilates ab curl is a very slow, careful movement, and it's important to concentrate on getting the right sensation to make sure that you are using your muscles correctly.

Lie on your back with your knees bent, feet hip-width apart. Place a folded towel between your knees and under your head. Rest your hands on your thighs. Relax your shoulders and breathe in. As you breathe out, draw your navel down towards your spine. Slide your hands up towards your knees and move your shoulder blades slightly down your back as you lift your upper torso and head off the floor. Curl your ribs forwards in the direction of your thighs, but don't feel you have to lift very far; a small lift is fine because you'll get most of the benefit from the first few centimetres of lifting. Repeat 10 times.

Caution: Did you feel any strain in your lower back? Be sure you don't start to curl until you can feel that your abdominals are engaged. Keep your neck soft and curl up from the abdomen; don't pull up with your head and shoulders.

Oblique curls

Lie on your back with your knees bent, feet hip-width apart. Place a folded towel between your knees, and another under your head. Place both hands beside your head and breathe in. As you breathe out, engage your abdominals and lift your right shoulder off the floor, moving it towards your left hip, keeping the left shoulder in contact with the floor. Pause, then breathe in as you curl back down again. Repeat 10 times on each side.

Variation: As you breathe out, engage your abdominals and curl your right shoulder towards your left hip, stretching your right hand past your left knee.

Caution: You shouldn't feel any strain in your neck as you curl upwards. Only start to curl when the abdominals are engaged. Keep your neck soft: avoid pulling up with your head and shoulders.

Hip rolls

This exercise also uses the abdominal muscles effectively. It is a good way of releasing any lower back tension.

Lie on your back with knees bent, feet hip-width apart and your knees together. Place a folded towel under your head. Relax your shoulders into the floor and place your hands on your abdominals to help you feel them stretch. Keep your back and neck long and relaxed. Breathe in, and as you breathe out, engage your abdominal muscles and move your knees to one side, keeping your buttocks glued to the floor and knees together. It's a very small movement and should be done very slowly. Repeat 10 times on each side.

Caution: If you have recently had a hip replacement, the inner thigh stretch and hip roll should be approached with caution.

Inner thighs

Sit on the floor with your back resting lightly against the wall. Making sure that your lower back touches the wall, spread your legs wide. Bend your right leg and hold the knee with your right hand. Flex your left foot. Breathe in and as you breathe out, engage your abdominals, and slide your left leg across the floor towards your bent right leg. Take it past the centre line (unless you have a hip replacement, in which case you should stop at the centre line). Breathe in to return to the starting position. Repeat 5 times on each leg.

Side twists

Sit upright on a chair or stool and touch your fingertips together in front of your breastbone, keeping your elbows lifted in line with your shoulders. Breathe in and as you breathe out, engage your abdominals, slide your shoulder blades down. Turn your upper body to the right, keeping your spine straight. Your arms should slide round softly and easily. When you have turned as far as you can go, pause. As you breathe out turn a little further and you'll feel an extra little stretch in the back. Breathe in and return to centre. Repeat 5 times in each direction in a smooth, continuous movement.

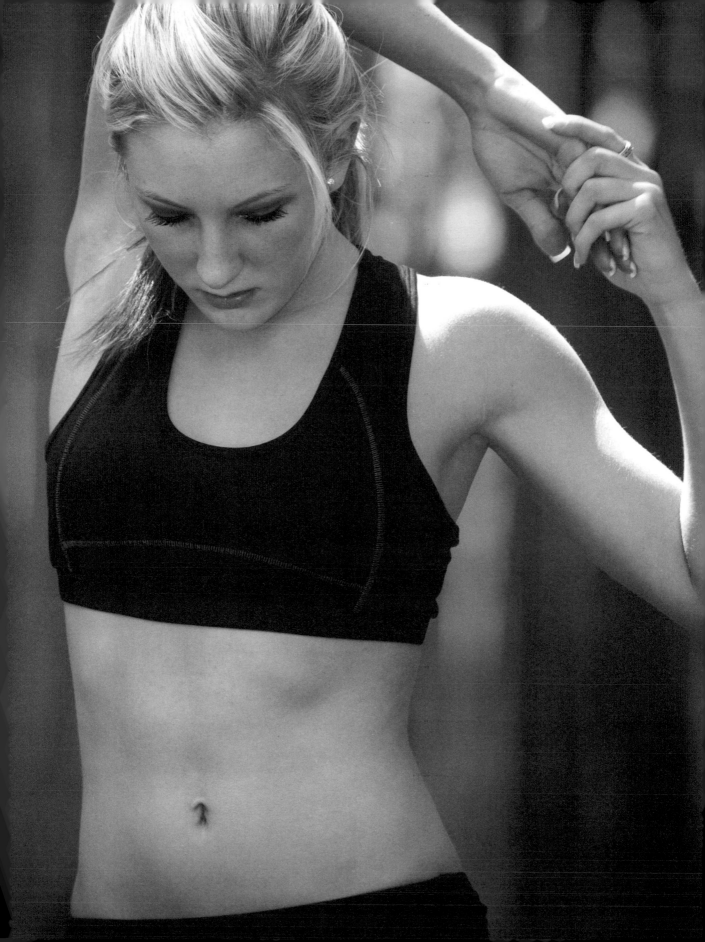

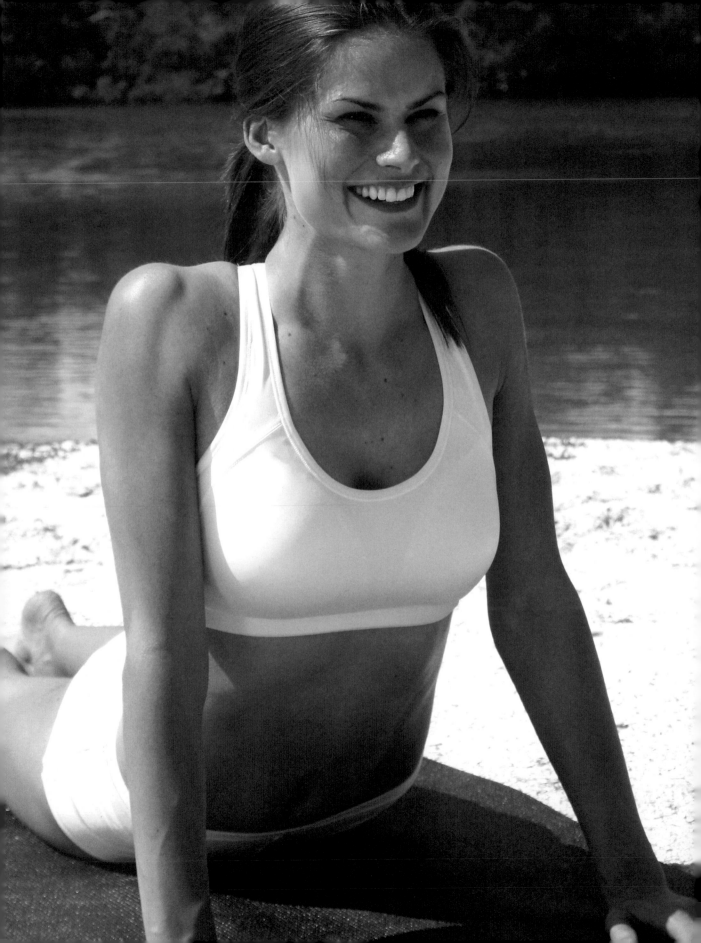

The better back programme

The price we humans pay for walking upright is that four out of five of us have a 'bad' back. Stretching and strengthening the muscles that support and stabilise your spine will protect you in the future by maintaining muscle balance and enhancing overall ease of movement. Integrate this core strength programme into your exercise routine twice a week, although it is advisable to consult your doctor before beginning if you have a back problem. Having a weak core is like building a home without a foundation. Use these core stabilisation and strengthening exercises to keep your back healthy. (You will see that there are abdominal exercises here, too. Remember the rule of symmetry: opposing muscles should be worked in tandem to prevent injury.) Yoga and Pilates will also focus heavily on the core region.

Always warm up beforehand.

Stabilisation exercises

Marching

- Preparation: lie on your back with your knees bent, feet hip-distance apart with your arms by your side. Now tighten up your abdominals and maintain this tension throughout the exercise whilst breathing naturally.

- Movement: lift one foot off the floor about 5cm while maintaining neutral spine and keeping the hips level. Slowly lower and repeat on the opposite leg. Repeat 10 times on each leg.

The plank

- Preparation: lie face down on the floor with your forearms underneath you so that you are supported on your elbows, and your elbows are directly below your shoulders.

- Movement: now tighten up your abdominal muscles, tense your buttocks and raise your hips just off the floor so you are supporting your body weight on your forearms and knees creating a straight line from your shoulders to your hips. Be careful not to let your hips sag so that your back arches. Similarly, do not raise your hips too high to make the exercise too easy. Hold your abdominals tight but breathe normally, maintaining this position for ten seconds before you relax back down. Repeat eight times.

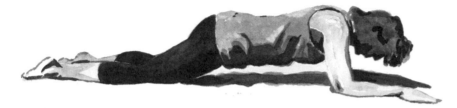

- Progression: start in the same position, but raise your entire body off the floor until it forms a straight line from head to toe, resting on forearms and toes.

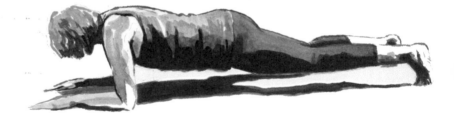

The prone cobra

- Preparation: lie face down on the floor with your arms beside your body, palms facing towards the ground.

- Movement: draw your navel in, tense your bottom and squeeze your shoulder blades together as you lift your chest and arms off the floor, pointing your thumbs to the ceiling. Hold for a few seconds and then slowly lower back to the start position. Keep the movement slow and control your breathing throughout. Avoid tilting the chin up and think about keeping your neck and head in line with your spine. Repeat eight times.

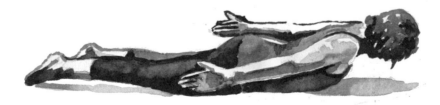

The swimming exercise

- Preparation: lie on your front resting your forehead on your hands, and keeping navel to spine and upper body relaxed.

- Movement: lengthen one leg away from the body before you lift it approximately 5cm from the floor. Keep the hips in contact with the floor and keep the movement slow and controlled. Breathe out as you lengthen and lift, breathe in as you lower the leg down. Repeat with the other leg. Always aim for length and not height. Repeat ten times on each leg.

- Progression 1 – alternating arm lifts: Lying on your front, raise your arms above your head in an open 'V' shape. Draw your navel towards your spine. Lengthen one arm away but focus on keeping the shoulder back from the ear, and raise the arm approximately 5cm from the floor, keeping the head in line with the arm, maintaining navel to spine. Slowly lower the arm and repeat the sequence with the other arm. Repeat 8 times with each arm.

- Progression 2 – alternating arm and leg lifts: keeping navel to spine, first lengthen and then raise the opposing arm and leg together approximately 5cm off the floor at equal height. Breathe out as you lift, keeping the hips in contact with the floor and navel to spine. Slowly lower and repeat with other arm and leg. Repeat 8 times on each side.

- Progression 3 – hands and knees: get on all fours and support yourself evenly, with your hands shoulder-width apart and your knees hip-distance apart. Ensure that your back is flat and your neck is in line with the spine. Breathe in, and as you exhale draw navel to spine without changing the alignment of the spine. Raise your right arm and left leg to a horizontal position. Hold briefly before returning your arm and leg to the start position. Repeat the sequence with your left arm and right leg. If balance is a problem, perform the leg movements and the arm movements separately. Repeat 8 times on each side.

Strengthening exercises

Curl-ups
Do between twelve and fifteen repetitions of the abdominal curls detailed in the summer section on page 118.

Obliques
To work the obliques, the muscles at the side of the waist, lie on your back, knees bent and feet hip-width apart. Raise one leg and place the ankle over the opposite knee. Place your opposite hand at the side of your head and rest the other arm at shoulder height on the floor. Breathe in and as you breathe out lift up and curl diagonally by rotating the shoulder (on the side where you are

supporting the head) towards the opposite hip. Remember to keep the elbow back, breathing out as you come up and in as you lower down. Repeat the exercise twelve to fifteen times, completing an equal number of repetitions on each side.

Back extensions
Do between twelve and fifteen repetitions of the back extensions detailed in the Summer section on page 119.

Flexibility exercises

To correct a muscular imbalance caused by poor posture or inactivity, remember that you need to not only strengthen the areas that are weak but also stretch those areas that are tight – tight muscles pull your spine out of alignment. Three areas in particular that need to be stretched in order to help prevent lower back problems are the hamstrings, hip flexors and glutes.

Hamstring stretch (back of thigh)
Lie on your back with knees bent and feet flat on the floor. Extend one leg up and hold it behind the thigh. Keeping your bottom in contact with the floor, bring the leg towards you until you feel a comfortable stretch at the back of the thigh, maintaining a straight leg. Hold for a minimum of twenty seconds and then repeat the stretch on the opposite leg.

Option: If you find it difficult to get hold of your thigh, wrap a towel around your leg and hold on to that instead.

Hip flexor stretch (front of hip)
Kneel down on one knee and take a big step forward with the other leg. Squeeze the buttocks on the side being stretched and gently press the hips forward until you feel a mild comfortable stretch in the hip area. The front knee should be bent at right angles i.e. with your knee in line with your ankle, behind the toes. Hold for a minimum of twenty seconds and then repeat the stretch on the opposite leg.

Option: Kneel on a towel or cushion for comfort if required.

Gluteal stretch (buttocks)
Sit up tall on the floor with your legs out straight. Bend your left knee and, keeping it upright, cross your left foot over and rest it to the outside of your right knee. Place your left hand beside your bottom and use your right hand to draw the knee in to feel the stretch. Now slowly turn your head to look over your left shoulder, and at the same time rotate your upper body toward your left hand and arm. This should increase your stretch. Hold for a minimum of twenty seconds. Repeat on both sides. Don't hold your breath, breathe easily.

Keep up aerobic exercise throughout autumn. It's been estimated that it only takes thirty minutes of cardiovascular exercise to mobilise white blood cells and kickstart them into action to remove invading germs.

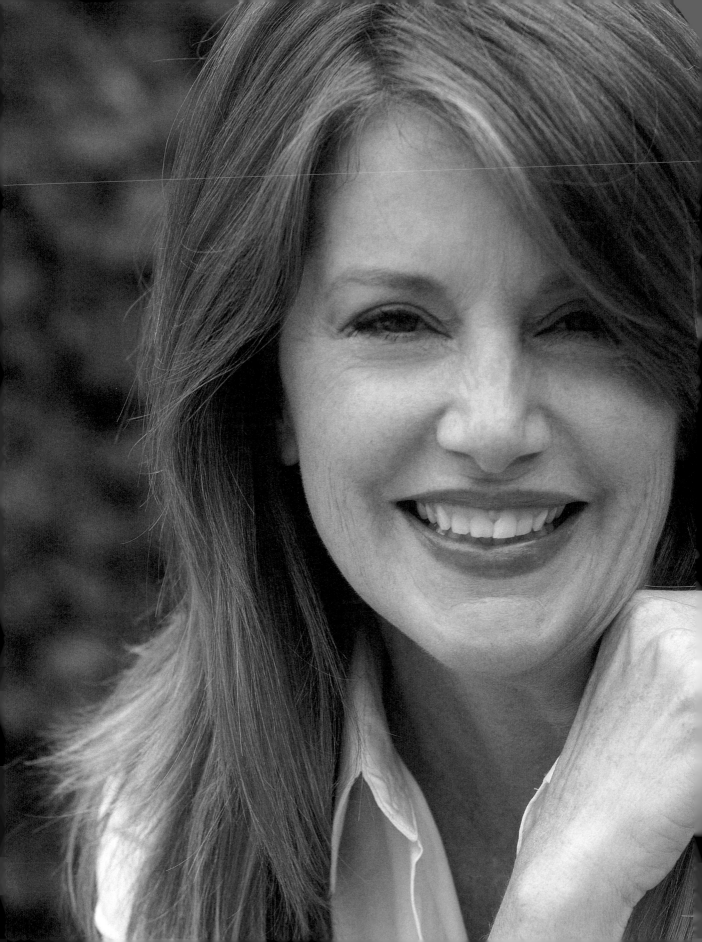

Love yourself

Autumn is the season for regaining your balance: skin and hair may need help adjusting to colder days; your sleep patterns may be thrown by the clock change in October; you may find it difficult readjusting to the stress of a faster pace after a languorous summer. The deeply relaxing treatments here have all been chosen because they help you achieve equilibrium, both physically and mentally.

Head in the Clouds

Let your mind unwind. A shoulder, neck and head massage will release tension and ease away the stress of the day. An oil and balm are applied for an intensive hair and scalp treatment.

You will need: oil such as Champneys Pure Relaxation Oil or follow the instructions in the Introduction for making your own; shampoo and conditioner.

Before you start: this works well seated as a DIY treatment but is even more relaxing if you can lie down and persuade a partner to treat you.

• Warm the oil in your hands and starting at the base of the neck, sweep your palms over your chest. Crossing your arms, move around the shoulders, down to the elbows and then back around the back of the shoulders to the back of the neck. Repeat, using your knuckles to knead the muscles.

• Rotate your head to the left and support it with your left hand. Press and rotate with the fingers of the right hand at the base of the skull where it meets the neck. Then make a fist and press the fist from the base of the skull over the shoulders and then back to the base of the skull. Gently rotate your head to the right and support it with your right hand, while you repeat the movement with your left hand on the left side.

• Warm more oil in your palms and apply it to the hair and scalp, right down to the ends of your hair.

• Rotate your head to the left, support it with the left hand and using the right hand, knead the back of your scalp with circular rotations. Then gently rotate your head to the right and support it with the right hand. Knead the back of the scalp with the left hand.

• Gently return your head to the centre and using both hands, massage the back of the head with circular rotations.

• Using both hands, knead your scalp with circular rotations, starting from the hairline towards the ears and then around the back of the head. Do this three times.

• Using the finger tips, starting at the hairline, apply pressure with each finger, circling with the hands but not the fingertips, release, and reapply working backwards from the hairline to the crown, and then to the ears and back to the base of the skull so that the whole head is covered. Leave an inch between each movement. ('Static spider circles' is the technical name and describes this movement well.) Do it three times.

• With a hand over each ear, move your fingers so that they slide towards the crown of your head. Work over the whole head this way, six times.

• With thumbs and forefingers, massage in circular movements up to the top of the ear and back down, then squeeze and pull each earlobe down three times.

• Using your palms, rotate the scalp using large static circles. Start from the hairline, move towards the ears and then around the back of your head. Do it three times.

• With both hands, gently lift sections of your hair and pull it in an outwards direction, then release the pull and take a new section of hair. Work towards the ears and around to the crown, and from there to the base of the skull.

• Starting at the hairline, rake your fingers through your hair until you reach the ends. Do this three times: the first time, firm; the second time, medium strength; the third time, lightly.

• Finish with a shower and shampoo, and condition your hair as normal.

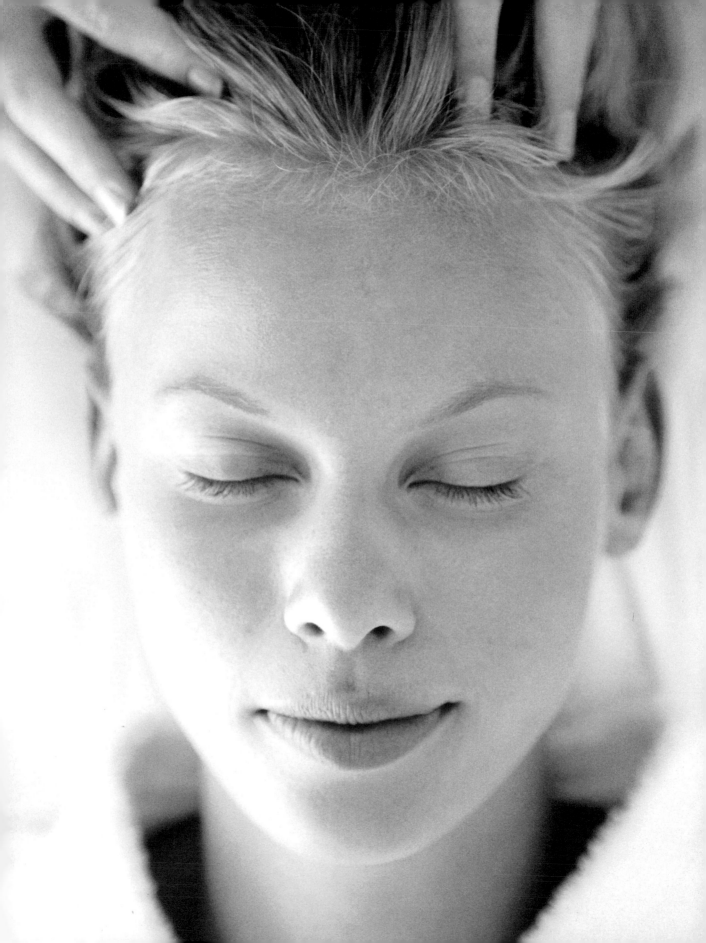

'Remember your hair needs a treat, too. Put on a conditioning hair treatment at the same time once a week as you put on a face mask. It saves time.'

Bed of Roses

This treatment involves rose-scented products and begins with a full body exfoliation followed by an application of body butter. You will then experience a relaxing wrap while the products do their magic. You will be left feeling cleansed, nourished and soothed by the gentle fragrance of the rose, which balances emotions and is deeply nourishing (incidentally, it is wonderful when your heart is hurt – rose traditionally heals an aching heart).

You will need: Champneys Skin Smoothing Rose Body Scrub and Champneys Ultra Rich Rose Body Butter plus base oil. You can make your own scrub by adding a few drops of rose essential oil and following the instructions in the Introduction.

Before you start: spread a blanket on your bed, or on a lounger or day bed. On top of it, place a clean linen sheet large enough to envelop your body. Have another blanket nearby and a pillow which will go under your head. An eye mask will help, or you could also use a silk scarf to block out the light while you relax.

Exfoliate

Stand in the bath or shower. Using large circular strokes, apply body scrub all over your body with vigorous brisk movements. Start with the back, chest and stomach. Then sweep from the tops of the feet to the thighs and from the back of the hands up the arms. Shower off the scrub in warm water (try Champneys Skin Softening Rose Body Wash).

Moisturise

Pat yourself dry with a warm towel and massage body butter thickly over your body.

Sit on the bed or lounger. Apply Champneys Intensive Cracked Heel Treatment Balm to your feet, or more of the body butter, and pop on some soft, cotton socks.

If your hair needs extra conditioning, follow the scalp massage movements from the previous treatment but using rose-scented oil. Wrap your head in a towel.

If your skin needs extra hydrating, apply Champneys Chamomile and Rose Moisture Miracle Mask or your own favourite. Apply Champneys Vitamiracle Rejuvenating Hand and Nail Cream or more body butter to your hands and pop on some cotton gloves.

Wrap and relax

Now wrap yourself as tightly as possible in the sheet and place the blanket on top. Put on your eye mask and lie back and relax for at least half an hour.

Take a nap if you can.

Afterwards, rinse the oil from your hair (if you used it), but don't shower your body – let the body butter sink in and replenish your skin's moisture levels.

Pure Balance Facial

This luxurious treatment uses a refining mud mask to remove surface impurities. It evens out the skin's complexion and provides silky smooth results for even the most tired-looking skin.

You will need a mud or clay mask to absorb excess oils and refine skin pores such as Champneys Cleanse and Purify Refining Mud Mask, toner, moisturiser, oil for a massage, a foamy cleanser and complexion brush or flannel, lip balm and an eye mask. A radiance-boosting product is optional.

Cleanse

Cleanse your face, eyes and lips as usual.

Use a foamy facial wash, such as Champneys Radiance Boosting Foamy Facial Wash, and a complexion brush or flannel to deep cleanse again.

Tone

Exfoliate using Champneys Natural Micro-Derm Facial Polish or similar product.

Tone once more.

Massage and masks

Massage your décolleté, shoulders, neck and face with Champneys Moisture Miracle Facial Oil or Super Rich Floral Facial Balm or a similar product.

Apply an eye mask with your index fingers such as Super Cooling Eye Rescue Gel, and then apply lip balm.

Apply a clay mask and leave it on for at least ten minutes while you relax.

Finish

Using damp cotton wool, sweep the eyes, lip and face to remove the products. Tone. Apply your usual moisturiser or a product designed to promote a radiant, firm complexion such as Champneys Perfect Skin Illuminating Beauty Balm.

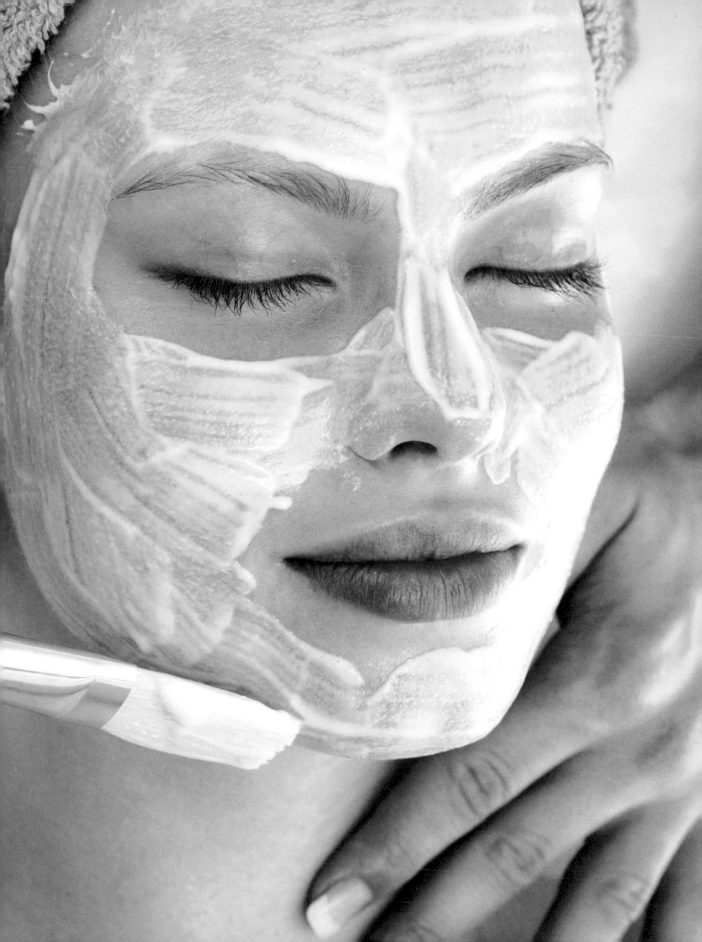

Take a power nap. If at all possible, a 10-minute nap between 2 and 4p.m. (even just resting with your eyes closed). Research has shown that this can increase alertness and productivity. (Longer than 20 minutes caused sluggishness.) It can also refresh you and make you feel happier about the rest of the day.

The Champneys 'sleep deep' plan

One in five of us are sleeping poorly, grabbing a few hours each night but waking unrefreshed, irritable and tired before the day even begins. Experts have coined a new term to describe this unsatisfactory state – 'junk sleep'.

Like junk food, junk sleep mimics the real thing but doesn't supply long-lasting sustenance. According to a recent survey, 46% of people said they typically got six hours or less each night, while 20% survived on less than five hours. Meanwhile, seven and a half hours is seen by experts as the minimum, and the latest research is nudging towards nine hours a night as the optimum. Without enough good quality sleep, it's impossible for us to be productive at work or stay on an emotional even keel. Sleeplessness might even be making us fat, as doctors report that those who sleep less than seven hours a night tend to be overweight. What is certain is that without sleep we age faster. One study found that when sleep was restricted to four to six hours, there were changes in hormone function that mimicked those that come with ageing.

We're not born with good sleeping habits. Babies have to be taught to go to sleep, and it is one of those lessons that some of us need to keep learning throughout our lives. Guests at Champneys find that the combination of an ultra-comfortable bed after a day involving movement, relaxation and fresh air, not to mention plenty of nutritious food, goes a long way to encouraging sleep. But if more help is needed, this bedtime ritual may help. Follow it religiously for a week.

Before you begin...

• Have zero tolerance of clutter. Your bedroom should be a peaceful sanctuary – free of mess, noise and anything pertaining to work. Lights should be soft. The floor and surfaces should be clear. Your bed should be inviting, with soft linens. Spray it with some lavender water or Champneys Perfect Sleep Pillow Mist.

• Pursue total darkness. Harvard research has shown that even the blinking of a standby light on a TV is registered through closed lids. Put up blackout curtains – street lights have been shown to keep people awake without them realising it. Switch off any hall lights.

- Restrict time in bed. Experts now think that associating bed with the agony of tossing and turning has psychological effects that stop people sleeping, so avoid that at all costs.

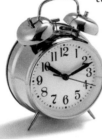

  - If you wake, and then lie awake for more than twenty minutes, get up and do something else. If you only sleep for five hours, set your alarm clock for the time you have to rise and go to bed five hours beforehand, even if that means staying up very late and getting exhausted. When you do go to bed, you will hopefully fall asleep easily. Next evening, go to bed fifteen minutes earlier and very gradually work back in increments of fifteen minutes until you are sleeping long enough. You'll know when that is if you wake refreshed and ready for the day ahead.

The plan itself

This assumes you intend to be asleep by 11 p.m. Adjust it to your bedtime accordingly.

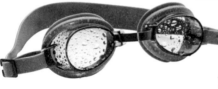

- 7 p.m. Around four hours before you go to bed, take a brisk walk, go for a swim or follow one of our core-strengthening routines for at least thirty minutes. Exercising in the early evening causes your parasympathetic nervous system to kick into gear, which slows your heart rate, blood pressure and breathing, signalling to your body that you're ready for sleep. Your body will start winding down even if you don't realise it.

- 8 p.m. With dinner, take 200–300mg of magnesium. This mineral helps the body make serotonin, which in turn produces melatonin, the brain chemical that sets your body 'clock'. Magnesium needs calcium for absorption, so take 400mg of calcium (it doesn't have to be at dinner).

- 9 p.m. Switch off the TV, computer, games console or any other screen. These stimulate your brain, making it harder to switch off later. Instead listen to the radio, some music or read a book. When your sleeping patterns are back on track, you may be able to watch a movie or favourite programme before bed and sleep well, but be aware that sleep experts think increased screen time is a main cause of sleeplessness, and it should always be monitored. If you are really serious about your sleep, switch on some gentle classical music. Research shows that those who listen to classical music before bed sleep better than those listening to any other kind.

• 9.30 p.m. Begin your 'before-bed' ritual. Lower the lights (or switch to candles). Rest on your bed or another quiet place in your home, shut your eyes and review your day. Let worries and doubts surface, resolve that you will deal with them tomorrow, and then allow them to float away. Consciously slow down your breathing and feel the tension leaving your body.

• 9.45 p.m. Run yourself a warm bath and add a soothing fragrance such as lavender or chamomile. This is a good time to indulge yourself with one of the treatments in this book as the concentration on yourself and your body will help to switch off worrying thoughts, as well as relax you. A warm bath triggers a reflex reaction that actually causes your body to try to cool itself down in response to heat. This cooling down is a powerful signal that it is time to sleep. For the same reason, ensure your bedroom isn't too hot. A slightly cooler bedroom will aid sleep.

• 10.30–10.45 p.m. It takes about fifteen minutes to fall asleep. Reading beforehand – nothing too stimulating! – should help. Novels written or set in the past are far more likely to soothe you to sleep than modern thrillers which remind you of the stresses and dangers of twenty-first-century life.

• 11 p.m. By now you should be drifting off to sleep. If not, stick with this programme. The secret – just as with little children – is total consistency.

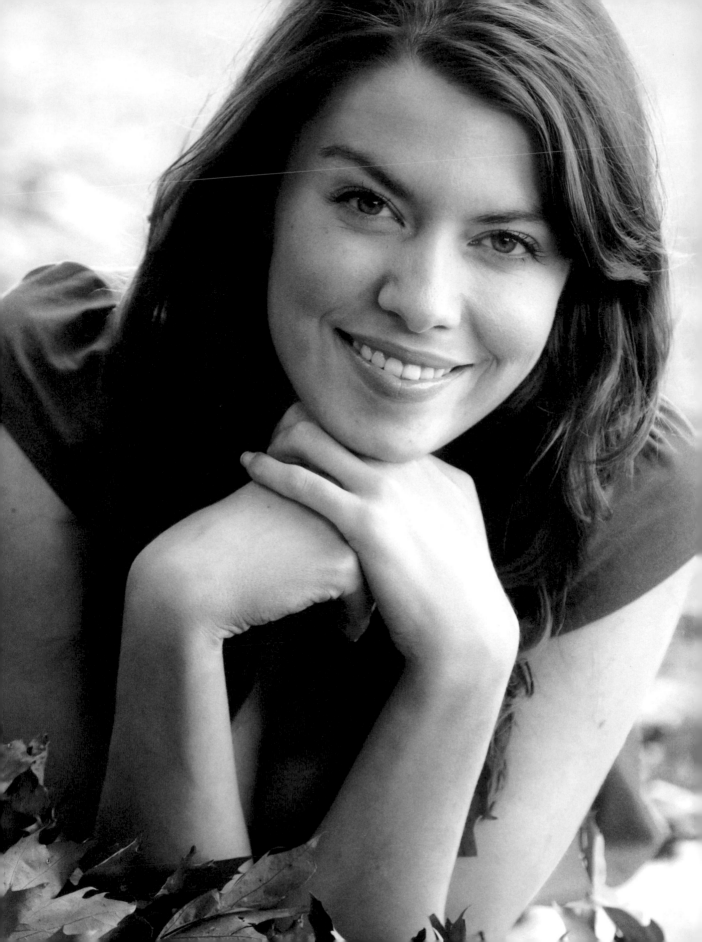

Well-being

Stress is disastrous for both sleep patterns and immunity, according to numerous studies. A recent survey discovered that two-thirds of Britons with poor sleep habits say that stress is the cause of their sleeplessness. This season, with its 'back to school' connotations, is a great time to tackle long-standing issues that have been causing you stress – like improving time management. Reclaim some time for yourself and you'll feel problems melting away as ennui, fatigue and listlessness – stress's close sisters – become a thing of the past.

Are you too busy to live your life?

Recreation is just that – the chance to recreate yourself. But so many of us are so busy that we never take time out. And the result is a 'flattening' of life, a feeling that we're losing out. We are: without the chance to recreate we lose our equilibrium, bounce and sparkle. Check yourself against these statements….

	Yes	No
1. You take a 'breather' every few hours during your working day.	☐	☐
2. Your personal life is unaffected by work.	☐	☐
3. You see plenty of the friends that matter.	☐	☐
4. You spend at least a small part of most days with someone who raises your spirits.	☐	☐
5. You have the space to act spontaneously at least once a week – catch a movie, watch the sunset, grab a cup of coffee with a friend on a whim.	☐	☐
6. You leave work at a reasonable time each day.	☐	☐
7. You always take all of your holiday allowance.	☐	☐
8. You always take a full hour for lunch unless there's a real emergency.	☐	☐
9. You always have time if a loved one needs half an hour.	☐	☐

Score one for every yes. Have you seven or more? You do have time for yourself and you probably feel there's enough time to follow your interests and come up with new ideas. With six or less, you need to slow down a little more to give your brain space to think.

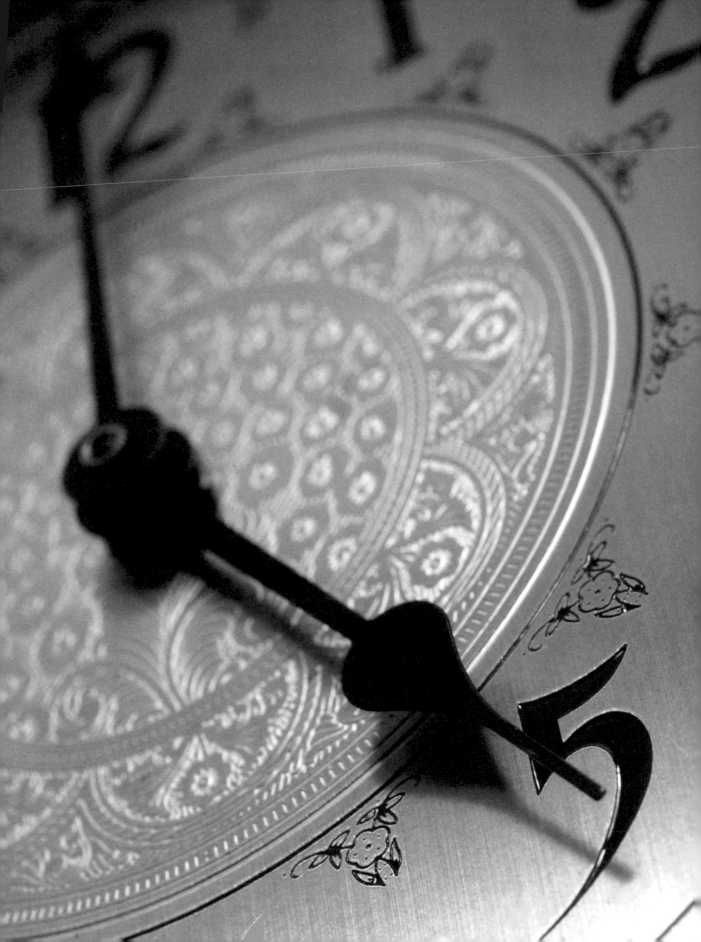

Take control of your time

Save time by following the tips below.

Leave work on time

Reduce interruptions and reclaim your evenings. Don't let your working day be hijacked by others. The secret is to have your goals clear in your mind. Think weekly, then daily. On Monday morning lose the sinking sensation that, 'I've got so much to do'. Instead, think 'What are my goals for this week?' Decide what you want to have done by Friday and then break each goal into smaller tasks that have to be undertaken to achieve all you want to do by Friday. Slot these tasks in throughout your week. This helps you prioritise, so that the tricky and difficult things or the tasks that depend on other people's input don't sink to the back of your consciousness. It also means you are giving attention to all that you have to do and not spending too much time on one task at the beginning of the week.

Never procrastinate again

Try the rotation method of time management, devised by life coach Mark Forster. Make a list of the top three tasks you have to complete this morning. Against each item write 10, 20, 30. These figures refer to blocks of minutes that you are going to spend on each item in turn. Start with the task that puts you off least. Set a kitchen timer or your mobile phone to go off in ten minutes. Do the task for ten minutes. After that period move on to the next task for ten minutes. Devote twenty, then thirty minutes to each task, sticking strictly to the alarm. If you finish one task, strike it from the list and flit between two tasks. This way you don't waste time postponing tasks you dread (any of us can do anything for just ten minutes) and you also work faster, because you know there is only limited time and a momentum is thus built into each task.

Give up the 'disease to please'

A huge amount of stress is caused by the inability to say 'no'. Result? We end up running to other people's agendas.

- Do you find yourself doing favours for others even when it doesn't suit you?
- Do you find yourself changing your own plans to fit in with other people's needs?
- Do you believe that if you stopped doing things for other people, they'd think less of you?
- Do you find yourself saying 'yes' when inside a little voice is screaming 'no, no, no'?

Answer 'yes' to any of these and it's time to stop falling into the approval trap. Think of some occasions where you find yourself agreeing to something you don't want to do. Practise in front of a mirror saying 'No, I'm afraid I can't'. The more you do it in private, the easier it becomes in 'real life'. Next, whenever you are asked to do something, make it a habit to say to yourself 'do I really want to do this?' rather than 'should I do this?'. If you don't want to do it, say 'no'.

Make time by trying out the following ideas.

Go where other people are

One study in Sweden showed that those who went to cultural events such as concerts, the cinema, plays and sporting events tended to live longer than their stay-at-home peers. The key factors could be increased social contact and reduced stress. Contact is key. The more ties you have to other people, the more likely you are to stay well in the first place. Researchers found that six or more connections to others made you four times better at fighting off the viruses that cause colds.

Have a good laugh

Researchers have found that the positive emotions associated with laughter decrease stress hormones and increase certain immune cells. Californian research found that an hour spent watching a funny programme significantly increased an important key hormone in the immune system. Invest in a boxed set of DVDs of your favourite sitcom or schedule lunch with friends who make you laugh. You should chuckle every day.

'What a wonderful life I've had! I only wish I'd realised it sooner.'

- COLETTE, WRITER

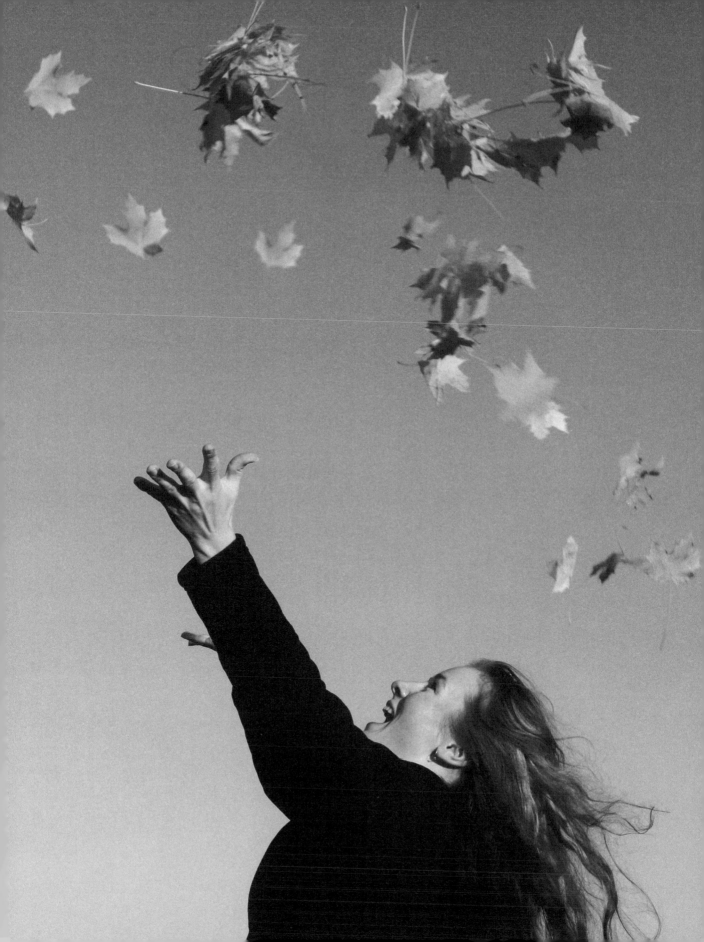

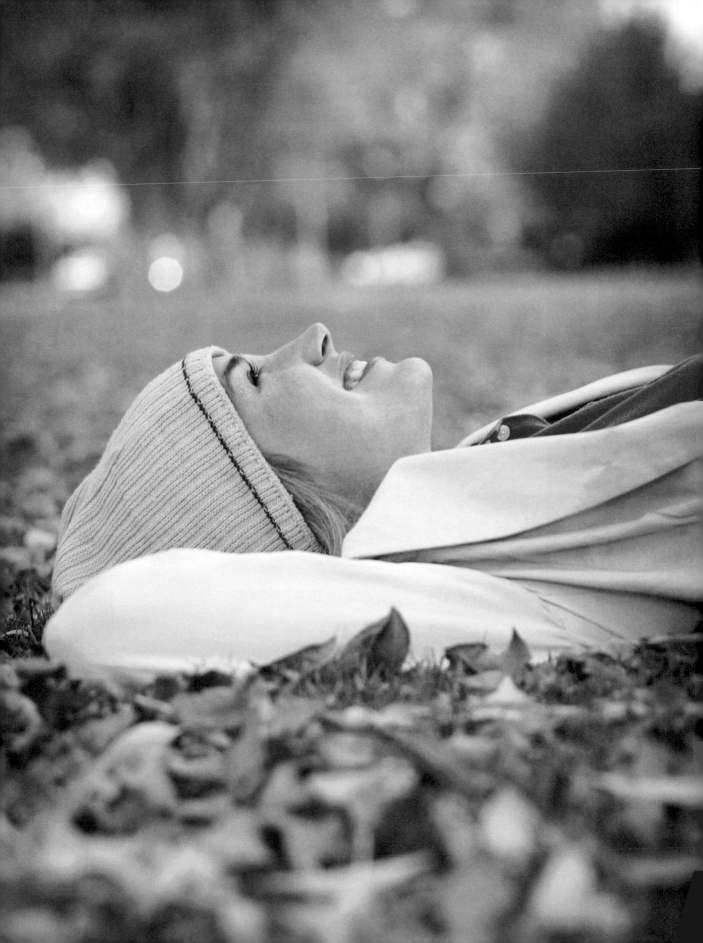

Escape – Be relaxed

Stress can motivate and challenge us but all too often overwhelm us. It can deplete energy and lead to anxiety, irritability and fatigue. The Champneys' Be Relaxed programme aims to relax and restore you while also helping you concentrate on what is draining your energy so you feel in control from now on. Through nutrition, exercise, massage and relaxation techniques we can help you maintain effective stress management. Here we've condensed the key factors of the programme into one day.

The Champneys restoration day

When you are facing burnout, or have been through a period of long-term chronic stress, book yourself a day out and follow this, your emergency recovery plan. You will feel rested, stronger and more in control in just twenty-four hours. Arrange for children to be looked after by others and ask your partner to forage for himself. The idea is that today you look after no one but yourself. Most importantly, don't reply to emails, and switch off your phone. The programme is based on three principles:

- Replenishing your body by giving it rest.
- Resting your brain by focusing on your body through gorgeous treatments and exercise.
- Nourishing your soul with healthy, simple food which will replenish the nutrients stripped out by stress.

On rising
Stay in bed. Stretch. Acknowledge that this day will be different. Today you are going to release tension. Do you feel like getting up? No? Then roll over and go back to sleep. When you do feel like getting up, prepare a mug of hot water with half a lemon squeezed into it and go back to bed. Read a favourite magazine or book. Take it easy. If you begin to feel guilty thinking of all you should be doing, breathe in for a count of eight and out for eight and tell yourself that if you burn out, you won't be able to do any of it.

217

Morning programme

Get dressed in comfortable clothes and go for a brisk twenty-minute walk. Listen to music or birdsong. Refuse to let annoying thoughts distract you. Breakfast on one of our inspirational breakfasts or simply chop a banana and a handful of nuts into some natural yoghurt. Have a

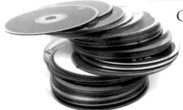

coffee or tea if you normally do. The last thing you want is withdrawal headaches from caffeine, but try to cut down on coffee and tea today – more than four cups a day makes you jittery even if you don't realise it.

After breakfast, indulge your body with a spa treatment. The 'Bed of Roses' on page 203 would work wonderfully.

Lunch

Try a tasty soup or lunch from our inspirational menus or have a huge salad combining every colour of vegetable you can think of. Dress with your favourite dressing. This meal must include one absolute treat – a glass of wine, a dish of ice-cream, a piece of chocolate. Enjoy.

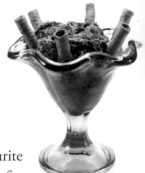

Afternoon programme

Go back to bed and sleep or read, or watch a favourite movie. A comedy will make you laugh – fabulous for stress levels. A weepie will make you cry – perhaps even better, if it serves as a cathartic release. Alternatively, lie on the sofa and listen to some favourite music. When was the last time you really listened to your music collection?

After some serious relaxing, aim for a few yoga or flexibility stretches. You do not have to be too serious about this. The idea is not so much to exercise but to notice where you are holding tension. Be curious as to why that is your stress reservoir. Work on releasing that tension. Become aware of all that your body does for you and how little you notice what is going on with it. Resolve that you will pay it more attention from now on.

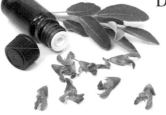

Dinner

Choose one of the recipes in this book for dinner and really enjoy preparing it. Put on some jazz if you like hip hop, disco if you prefer classical. Mix things up… dance to a different rhythm. Don't rush the preparation or the meal. Enjoy it by candlelight.

Before bed

Enjoy a long candlelit soak with scented oils – if you have the time and energy, indulge in a facial or relaxing foot massage (wonderfully grounding). Resist the temptation to watch TV – it will ruin the mood. Go to bed early. Read a book or listen to some classical music. Drift off to a sound sleep.

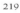

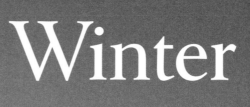

Winter

Five ways to celebrate winter

• Reach out. On cold mornings, roll over for a cuddle as the best possible start to the day. Levels of oxytocin, the bonding hormone, are high when we wake at around 7–8 a.m. (for both sexes). Or email a child who has left home or a good friend at the other side of the world so their day gets off to a good start, or write a quick card of appreciation to a loved one. Harness those loving feelings and send them out before your day is hijacked by other emotions, other hormones.

• Celebrate with candlelight. The winter equinox is 21 December, the traditional Festival of Lights. From now on, the darkness recedes. Celebrate by lighting candles all round the house, firing up fairy lights and having some friends round for a pre-Christmas drink.

• Make a wish list. Ask all family members to write down what they want from the year ahead, pop the lists in an envelope, mark it with next year's date and pop it in when you're packing away the Christmas decorations. It will give you something to talk about next Christmas and is a fascinating keepsake of your family's journey.

• Supercharge your skincare routine. Now is the time to indulge in facials and lavish extra care on your skin. Think about introducing facial oil, such as Champneys Super Rich Floral Facial Balm, to your routine for extra moisture.

• Relax as you heal. Aromatherapy oils are lightning fast mood- and stress-relievers, and in this potentially frantic period, learning quick ways to use them is a wise strategy. For example, add some revitalising pine fragrance to a foot bath after a heavy day Christmas shopping. Fill a bowl with warm water, add five drops of soothing German chamomile, rinse a facial cloth in the water and spread it over your clean face while you have a quick lie down. (You could put two used chamomile teabags over your eyes to heighten the effect and wake up tired eyes.)

The season of joy and peace

December is a great month to luxuriate in warming treatments that restore energy levels – book a floatation or a hot stone massage.

January is a great month to retreat. Take a few days out for yourself to fine-tune your health and rest to recover from the party season. Check out page 285 for our Be Revitalised programme.

February is a great month to spread the love. Don't take your partner for granted. Focus some extra love and attention on your partner all month and you might be surprised by the results. But on Valentine's Day, don't just make it about him. Send cards to everyone who is special to you – it will make their day.

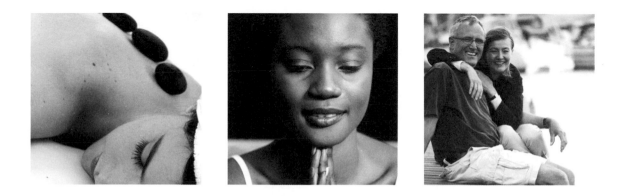

December... January... February... Winter

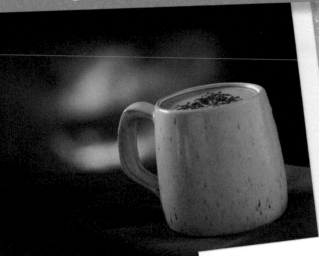

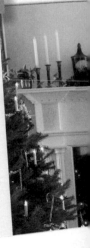

Restore... your spirit on quiet, snowy winter nights; time to draw closer to the fire and dream.

Comfort... yourself with warming soups, laughing with friends, the thrill of Christmas Eve (always new, always the same).

Rediscover... your favourite cashmere cardi; a younger-looking you; love.

Unwind... with spirit-enhancing yoga; warming, soothing treatments; brisk walks on frosty mornings.

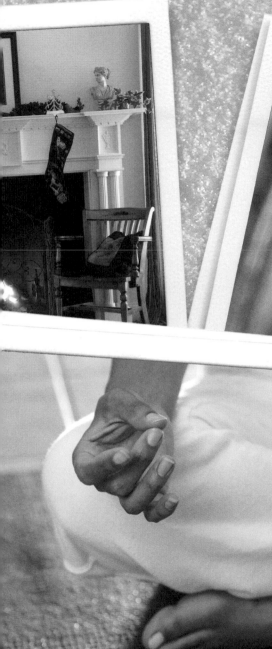

Release... tension from your shoulders, lines from your face — and your inner artist.

Reconnect... with who and what truly matters.

Eat

Live longer, look better, be healthier. You can increase the length of your life by an astounding fourteen years with just two simple measures:

- Follow the nutritional and exercise guidelines in this book (in other words, eat healthily, exercise moderately).

- If you smoke, give up.

It's not just length of life but also quality of life that can be improved by a healthy lifestyle. Making these changes means you will stay slimmer, be more mobile, more energetic and, yes, more youthful for years longer than your peers.

A key component of an anti-ageing diet is to beat free radicals. Free radicals are particles that attack the body's cells, and can damage or kill them. They're a by-product of normal body processes, like making energy, but also produced by smoking, sun damage, stress, alcohol and a poor diet. (Now you know why these things all make you look years older. The more damage you are exposed to, the more free radicals you produce.) Free radicals bombard healthy cells, damage DNA and mitochondria and contribute to cancer and heart disease. Free radical damage is a major cause of ageing. Antioxidants – vitamins, minerals and other nutrients – fight free radicals, which is why those of us who eat more of them look and feel younger.

Are there any other important anti-ageing factors? Well, eat regular, modest meals, including breakfast, and avoid sugar and refined or processed grains. Blood-sugar stability has a key role in anti-ageing. Unbalanced blood-sugar levels result in increased 'glycosylation' (sugar molecules binding to proteins, disrupting normal function). This, in turn, results in ageing and ill-health. It also affects insulin production which can lead to weight gain. Aim for four or five mini-meals a day or three meals and two snacks.

Is it worth taking a supplement?

Food isn't what it used to be – and neither are our diets. RDAs (Recommended Daily Allowances – referred to on food packaging) were established as levels to prevent disease – not to achieve optimum health. Most RDAs assume that you are in good health, stress-free, under the age of sixty, and have a good digestion so you can absorb the nutrients in food perfectly.

Many experts consider a multivitamin supplement to be a good idea. Harvard researchers reported in 2002 that 'most people do not consume an optimal amount of vitamins by diet alone' and concluded that in view of 'strong evidence of effectiveness' from controlled trials, 'it appears prudent for all adults to take vitamin supplements.'

When choosing a formula for anti-ageing, make sure it contains good levels of B vitamins, including folic acid. An important indicator for lifespan (and healthspan) is how much homocysteine you accumulate. Homocysteine is a toxic protein that is a by-product of body reactions, and is usually transformed into beneficial substances. But it needs certain conversion factors to make this possible: vitamins B6, B12, folic acid and betaine. Without enough of these, homocysteine builds up. Low homocysteine levels in the blood are important for our good health. (You can get a DIY blood test from York Testing to check your own levels at home.) Betaine is especially effective at reducing homocysteine levels; top betaine-containing foods include spinach, eggs, freshwater shrimps and prawns.

Consider a coenzyme Q10 supplement – you probably won't find this in a multivitamin formula. After the age of twenty, natural production of coenzyme Q10 slows down – and by forty, it's at a quarter of its original level. Every cell in your body needs coenzyme Q10 for repair, so good levels are essential if you want to continue looking youthful. Eat lots of broccoli, cabbage and Brussels sprouts, which help increase Q10's effectiveness in your body, and consider a supplement as it's hard to get enough from food.

With a little help

These people may need some extra help to meet micronutrient requirements...

- Anyone who is pregnant or breastfeeding. Increased needs: B vitamin family, folic acid, vitamins D and probably E, and minerals like iron, magnesium, calcium. Take a supplement designed for pregnancy.

- Post-menopausal women. Increased needs: extra calcium, magnesium and supporting minerals for bones, and vitamins A, B, C, D, E and K.

- Women on the Pill. Taking the Pill is thought to increase the need for folic acid, vitamins B and C and zinc.

- Sunbathers. Sun uses up antioxidants. Increased needs: vitamins A, C and E – and also increase your carotenoid and flavonoid intake.

- Dieters. Reducing food intake reduces micronutrient intake, but the need for some vitamins and minerals can rise. Anorexics and bulimics also risk multiple micronutrient deficiency.

- Vegetarians/vegans. The overall diet requires careful thought. There could be a shortfall of vitamins D and B12, iron, zinc, omega 3 fats and complete proteins. Animal proteins contain all the essential amino acids; most plant-derived proteins do not. But you can get all of them by eating a balanced mix of plant-based proteins, for example, by combining grains and pulses.

- Smokers. Smokers need to be cautious about supplementing with beta-carotene – it can be dangerous. Smoking depletes the body of vitamin C so intake should be increased.

- Anyone who has had an accident, illness or surgery. Increased needs: many vitamins and minerals, including calcium, zinc and magnesium; vitamins A, B, C and E.

- Older people. Digestion becomes less efficient with age and multiple micronutrient depletion is very common. A good multivitamin/mineral programme is even more important for anyone over sixty.

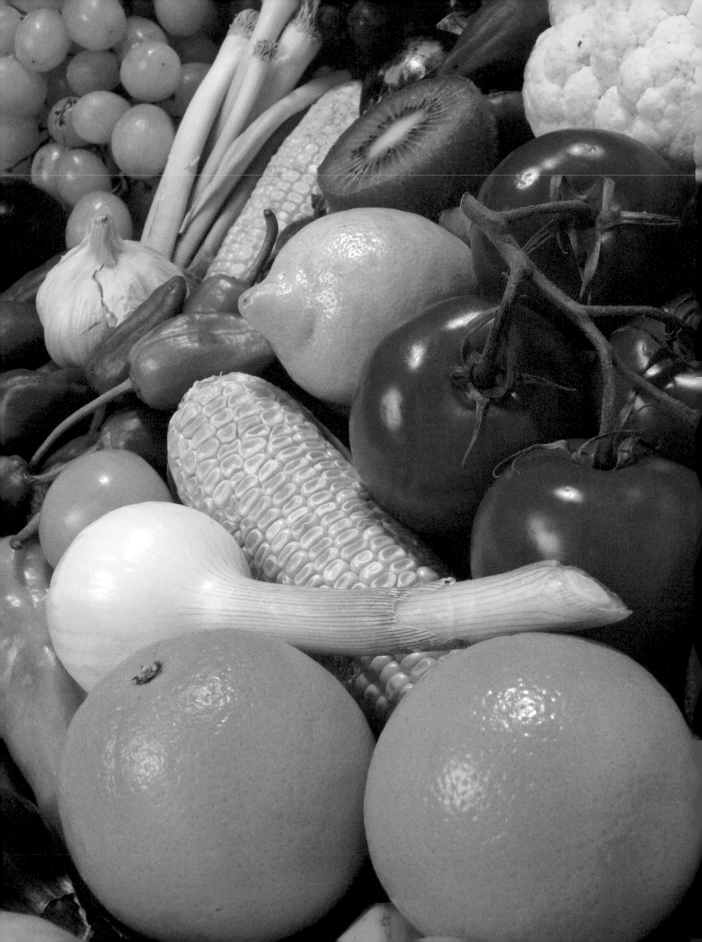

The anti-ageing shopping list

Antioxidants are the key to anti-ageing. These are the foods that provide them in beneficial quantities.

Lots of vegetables and fruit

The first priority in fighting the signs of ageing is to increase fruit and vegetable intake to a minimum of nine portions a day. Five servings a day is the bare minimum: UK intake was so low that it was thought that this was a reasonable start point to aim for when the guidelines were drawn up, but those who are serious about their health – like some cancer experts – aim for double this amount.

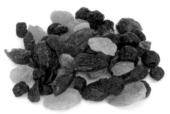

Thinking in terms of whole fruits and spoonfuls of vegetables, nine can seem daunting – but think 'how do I supersize the antioxidant content in everything I eat?' instead. For instance, toss a handful of dried fruit onto cereal and into yoghurt; snip some curly kale or raw broccoli over salads and into soups; open your lunchtime sandwich and grate carrot over it; pop in half a dozen cherry tomatoes as you make a cheese omelette.

Sufficient protein

Protein promotes cellular repair and growth. Healthy protein sources are foods such as poultry and game, seafood, legumes and traditional soya foods (though you may want to choose organic – a lot of soya production is genetically modified).

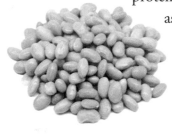

Brown rice

Brown rice is a good source of thiamine (vitamin B1). This B vitamin slows down the stiffening of collagen fibres and helps prevent wrinkles. If your skin looks tired and you have dark circles, you may well be lacking in vitamin B1 because it is crucial for a healthy circulation. It is also easily broken down by smoking and alcohol. Brewer's yeast, available in supplement form, is a particularly rich source of vitamin B1.

Nuts and olives

Cashews, walnuts and olives are sources of copper – and low copper levels can lead to premature greying. Eating foods rich in copper (the best sources are liver and shellfish) improves melanin production, and that's the pigment which supplies the colour in hair. Try to eat a source of copper most days.

Seaweed

Nori and wakame seaweeds are rich in selenium, amongst other minerals, which works with vitamin E to combat premature signs of skin ageing. It's estimated that our bread, for instance, contains about 50% less selenium than it did fifty years ago because of degradation of the soil, so looking to the sea for selenium makes good sense.

Iron-rich foods

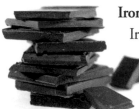

Iron is essential for energy and healthy hair and skin, but menstruation depletes iron stores, so iron deficiency is common in pre-menopausal women. Non-red meat iron needs help from vitamin C to be absorbed, so eat some fruit or green vegetables alongside other iron-rich foods such as seafood, dried fruit, dark chocolate and wholewheat.

Green tea

Three or four cups of green tea a day will give you a powerful boost of antioxidants, as well as supplying fluid. Drinking plenty of water helps plump up the skin and eradicate fine lines. Drink a glass of water one hour, and a cup of green tea the next and carry on throughout the morning. Green tea contains caffeine, so might affect your sleep if you drink it later in the day.

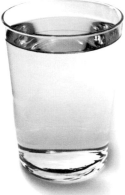

Lessons to be learned

The Hunza people of the Himalayas are some of the longest-lived in the world and famous for their natural vigour and energetic ways. Why? It's thought that one reason is due to a diet loaded with foods which happen to be high on the oxygen radical absorption capacity (ORAC) scale. This scale, developed by scientists at the prestigious Tufts University in the USA, measures the antioxidant content of foods. Eating foods with a high ORAC score will increase blood antioxidant levels by up to 25%. So pass the prunes, raisins, blueberries, kale, spinach and red kidney beans (not just for chilli con carne). As a rough guide, the deeper the colour the higher the ORAC (so think kale rather than lettuce).

The people with the longest healthy lifespans live on Okinawa, an archipelago of islands off Japan. They eat small portions and it is a way of life for them never to over eat – 'Eat until you're 80% full' is their mantra. Animal research shows that calorie restriction slows ageing and we know that the health costs of being overweight are very real. Opt for moderation.

Both the Okinawans and the Hunzas eat less meat than we do in the West. This is no coincidence. Vegetarians eating a good diet can live on average ten years longer than carnivores; some research shows a good vegetarian diet can reduce your risk of dying from cancer by 40%, and of developing heart disease by 30%. Eat meat sparingly. Instead choose plenty of fish, lentils and beans, grains like quinoa and bulgur, eggs, yoghurt, cheese, nuts and seeds, plenty of vegetables and a good amount of fruit.

Herbs

Oregano has twenty times the antioxidant activity as most other herbs. So pop some in your trolley and add it to tomato-based sauces, sprinkle it over pizza or grilled meat and toss a pinch into soups. Lots of other herbs and spices have anti-ageing abilities too, including rosemary, thyme, garlic, turmeric and ginger.

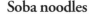

Soba noodles

Made from buckwheat, which is related to the rhubarb family and a good source of the flavonoids quercetin and rutin, soba noodles are a great alternative to less nutritious egg noodles. Changing the water half way through cooking cuts down on the chance of the noodles sticking.

Nut butters

Nut butters are good for you. Almond butter is usually less salty than peanut butter and can be substituted for butter in sandwiches. Almonds are also a good source of both vitamin E and monounsaturated fat, also known as omega 9, which help protect the heart.

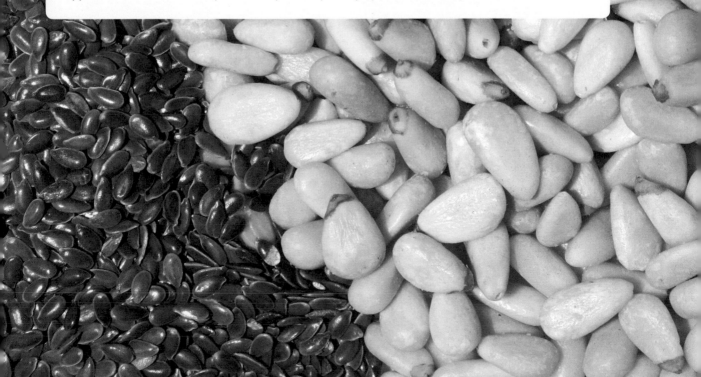

Ailsa Higgins, Champneys' Nutritionist, says: *'The fats and oils in your diet have a big impact on how well you age. Our bodies recognise and need natural fats. Big troublemakers are man-made hydrogenated or partially-hydrogenated fats which produce trans fats – an ageing nightmare. They're associated with increased free-radical damage to cell membranes, triggering inflammation, disease and degenerative processes. Read food labels and avoid those containing 'hydrogenated' or 'partially-hydrogenated' fats. Keep the amount of saturated fat in your diet low: use butter sparingly and substitute olive oil (dip bread in it rather than spread it with butter or magarine) and include nuts also seeds, flaxmeal and oily fish in your diet. Consider a fish oil supplement because that may well add years to your lifespan and healthspan.'*

Are you an emotional eater?

When is food not food? When you get it mixed up with your best friend and expect it to support you when you're feeling down, that's when. This is especially true in winter and this is a good time to work out if you eat solely for hunger or look to food for comfort. Tick the relevant boxes.

	rarely	sometimes	often
1. I eat when I'm not hungry…	☐	☐	☐
2. I often think about my next meal when I've just eaten…	☐	☐	☐
3. When I'm feeling low, food 'calls' to me and I can't think of anything else until I eat it…	☐	☐	☐
4. I'm always starting a new diet…	☐	☐	☐
5. …but even as I start I know I won't keep to it.	☐	☐	☐

How did you score?

Three or more 'Rarely': you have a healthy attitude to food most of the time and see it for what it is – fuel.

Three or more 'Sometimes': you have an ambivalent attitude to food and turn to it to fulfil emotional as well as physical needs. Ask yourself what emotion you're looking to satisfy when you find yourself making bad nutritional choices, and then think of another way that satisfaction could be met.

Three or more 'Often': You are a comfort eater and look to food to lift you when you're down. This probably causes you distress because at best your emotional needs are not being met, at worst your eating habits are affecting your physical health, too. You may benefit from some counselling around the issues of food to explore where you learned to use food in this way and change your attitude towards it.

'If you find yourself craving something sweet or starchy, eat something protein-rich – fish, cheese, meat, eggs – instead. This will balance your blood sugar and get you off the rollercoaster that perpetuates the craving cycle. A boiled egg can make a good mid-morning or afternoon snack. People are still worried about the cholesterol eggs contain but studies don't substantiate a link between egg-eating and heart disease. Eating one egg a day is unlikely to affect the heart-disease risk in healthy men and women.'

– AILSA HIGGINS, CHAMPNEYS' NUTRITIONIST

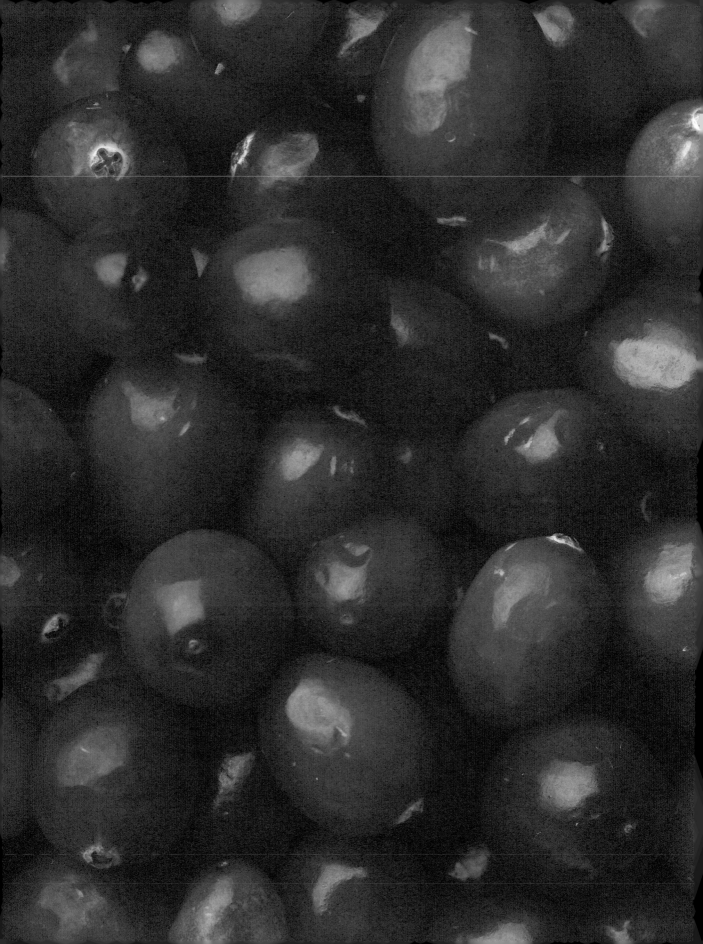

Inspiration to eat well...

Breakfasts

Traditional Scottish porridge
(serves 4)
150g oatmeal
500ml soya milk
250ml water
A small pinch of salt

Place the oatmeal in a thick-bottomed saucepan and cover it with the milk and water. Add the salt. Gently heat it through and simmer for 10 minutes. Then spoon the porridge into warm bowls and serve immediately. Plain porridge can also be served with honey or dried fruits (omit the salt), or try sprinkling some sunflower and pumpkin seeds on top.

Christmas cranberry, blood orange and pomegranate juice
(serves 1)
5 blood oranges
100g fresh cranberries
2 pomegranates
Honey – optional, to taste
Cinnamon, to serve

A citrus press works well here. Extract the juice from all the fruit and blend it together. Taste the result and add honey if required to counteract the natural bitterness of the fresh cranberries. Serve with a pinch of cinnamon.

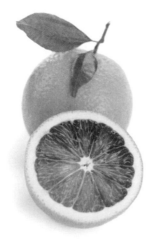

This recipe is high in vitamin C, great for immunity and in helping to absorb iron. Pomegranates and cranberries are high on the ORAC scale (see page 233), which is linked to antioxidant protection. Blood oranges and pomegranates also contain some minerals including modest amounts of potassium, calcium and iron. These important nutrients support bone and joint health, and the nervous system – and help regulate heart function.

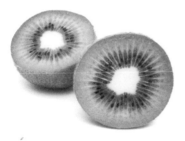

Vitamin smoothie

(serves 1)

1 banana, peeled and chopped

1 orange, peeled and chopped

2 kiwi fruit, peeled and chopped

100g frozen mixed berries

100ml pomegranate juice

100ml orange juice

Put all the ingredients in the blender and whizz them together. Serve immediately.

Pomegranate is a 'superfood', packed with antioxidants which support a healthy heart and have anti-ageing properties, protecting cells from free-radical damage. Oranges, kiwis and berries are all rich sources of vitamin C which supports the immune system and firms the skin. Unripe bananas provide special fibre that helps protect the gut wall and feeds healthy gut bacteria, which are vital for supporting your digestion and encouraging stable blood sugar.

Smoked haddock kedgeree

(serves 2)

1 egg

250ml water

100g brown basmati rice

150g smoked haddock fillet

Enough semi-skimmed milk to cover the fish

A handful of chopped parsley

Paprika, to serve

First, hard-boil the egg and place it in cold water to cool. Then cook the rice: put 250ml water in a pan and bring it to the boil. Add the rice, stir and cover the pan with a lid. Reduce the heat and cook the rice for about 20 minutes until all the water is absorbed. After the rice has been cooking for about 12–15 minutes, place the fish in a small pan and cover it with milk. Simmer it slowly for about 6 minutes, depending on the thickness of the fillet. Peel and chop the hard-boiled egg. Remove rice from the heat, drain any remaining liquid and fluff it up with a fork. Quickly flake the smoked haddock and add it to the rice with the chopped egg and the parsley. Stir everything together gently and serve immediately – sprinkle with a little paprika if you wish.

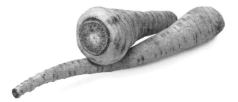

Lunches and main courses

Parsnip, honey and mustard soup

(serves 4)

500g parsnips, peeled and chopped

2 onions, chopped

1 leek, chopped

3 sticks celery, chopped

2 garlic cloves, chopped

½ tsp crushed coriander seeds

2 bay leaves

750ml vegetable stock

150ml semi-skimmed milk

1 tsp wholegrain mustard

1 tsp honey

Juice of half a lemon

Salt and pepper

1 tbsp chopped parsley, to serve

Put the parsnips, onions, leek, celery, garlic, coriander seeds and bay leaves in a thick-bottomed saucepan, add the stock and cook for about 20–30 minutes until all the vegetables are tender. Remove the bay leaves, then liquidise the soup. Pour it into a large bowl and add the milk, mustard, honey and lemon juice. Season to taste with salt and pepper, then pass it through a sieve. Put it in a clean pan and reheat it gently, then serve sprinkled with the chopped parsley.

> Parsnip is one of the foods highest in soluble fibre, which lowers cholesterol and blood pressure. Parsnip also contains around half a dozen potent antioxidants.

Saffron, potato and garlic broth

(serves 4–6)

1 tbsp olive oil

½ tsp chopped oregano

6–8 garlic cloves

125ml white wine

900g new potatoes, peeled and sliced

1 litre fish stock

A pinch of saffron strands

Heat the olive oil in a heavy-bottomed saucepan and add the oregano and cloves of garlic, and cook for a few minutes until the garlic is very slightly brown. Remove from the heat, allow to cool slightly, then add the white wine and reduce until this has completely evaporated. Add the sliced potato with the stock and the saffron, cover with a lid and simmer for 15–20 minutes until the potatoes are tender. Serve immediately.

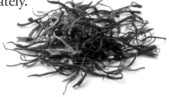

241

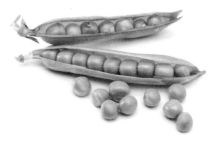

Pan-fried scallops with a pea purée

(serves 4 as a starter, 2 as a main course)

25g butter

250g frozen peas

100ml chicken stock

Salt and pepper

12 scallops, cleaned

A little sunflower oil

Mixed salad leaves, to serve

Balsamic vinegar, to serve

Put the butter, peas and stock in a pan and simmer for 3–4 minutes. Transfer them to a blender and whizz them together briefly to make a purée. Check it for seasoning, adding salt and pepper if necessary, then return the purée to the pan and keep it warm over a very low heat; don't allow it to catch.

Season the scallops. Heat a little sunflower oil in a non-stick pan until very hot, then sear the scallops on both sides for about 1 minute. Put a bed of purée on each plate, and place the scallops on top. Quickly toss the salad leaves with some balsamic vinegar and put them on the plates, next to the scallops. Serve immediately.

Sliced fig, Parma ham and Gorgonzola salad

(serves 2)

4 ripe figs

100g Gorgonzola cheese, diced

2 small of bunches watercress

6 slices of Parma ham

For the dressing:

2 tbsp olive oil

1 tbsp balsamic vinegar

Make the dressing – whisk the balsamic vinegar and olive oil until they emulsify, or shake them together in a firmly sealed clean jar. Arrange two figs, half the cheese, three slices of Parma ham and some watercress on each plate, drizzle with the dressing and serve immediately.

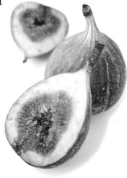

Figs help promote bowel regularity. They also provide a good helping of minerals and are one of the richest plant sources of calcium.

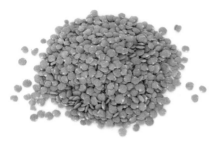

Lentil dhal

(serves 4–6)

1 onion, finely diced

1 carrot, finely diced

1 leek, finely sliced

2 sticks celery, finely diced

2 garlic cloves

600ml vegetable stock

1 tsp turmeric

A pinch of garam masala, ground ginger, ground coriander, ground cumin, chilli powder and paprika

200g red lentils, rinsed

Salt and pepper to taste

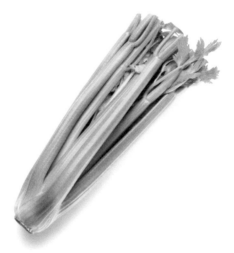

Place all the vegetables and the garlic in saucepan with 2–3 tbsp of vegetable stock and cook over a medium heat until softened. Then add the spices and heat for 1–2 minutes. Now add the lentils and heat for a further 1–2 minutes until all the moisture is absorbed, then cover with the rest of the vegetable stock, season with salt and pepper and cook for 30–45 minutes until the lentils are softened and all the stock has been absorbed. Check during this time to make sure that the lentils are not catching; add a little water if necessary. Once cooked, serve with brown basmati rice.

Dhal can be eaten on its own as a healthy and filling dish, and is great for people trying to lose weight.

Lentils contain valuable minerals, including iron (eat with foods rich in vitamin C, such as tomatoes, peppers and broccoli, to promote absorption). They're also a great source of folic acid, an essential nutrient often lacking in Western diets.

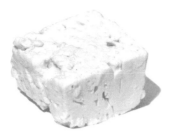

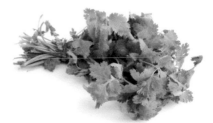

Butternut squash, feta cheese and parsley patties

(serves 2)

300g cooked butternut squash

100g feta cheese, diced

A handful of parsley, chopped

A little flour, for dusting

A little olive oil

Mixed salad leaves, to serve

Greek yoghurt, to serve

Roughly mash the cooked butternut squash. In a bowl, mix the mashed squash, diced feta and chopped parsley together well. Shape the mixture into two patties. Put them on a plate and dust them with a little flour, then turn them over and sprinkle the flour on the other side. Chill them in the fridge for 30 minutes. Heat a little oil in a non-stick pan and remove the patties from the fridge. Using a broad flat tool like a fish slice, gently put both the patties into the pan and fry them for 5 minutes, turning them carefully, until golden brown. Serve with mixed leaves and a spoonful of Greek yoghurt on the side.

Chicken tagine with sweet potato, carrots and prunes

(serves 4)

1 tbsp olive oil

12 small button onions

2 sweet potatoes, peeled and diced

2 carrots, diced

1 tbsp grated ginger

Ground black pepper

12 prunes, stones removed

1 tsp ground cinnamon

1 tsp honey

375 ml chicken stock

4 chicken breasts, each cut into 4 pieces

½ tbsp chopped coriander

½ tbsp chopped mint

Pre-heat the oven to 170ºC / gas mark 4. Heat the oil and gently cook the onions until soft and golden, add the sweet potatoes, carrots and ginger, season with a little black pepper and cook until the vegetables start to colour slightly. Stir in the prunes, cinnamon and honey and allow them to heat through, then add the chicken stock. Put the chicken breasts in a deep roasting tray, pour the vegetables over them and cook in the oven for 30–40 minutes. Stir in the coriander and mint, and serve.

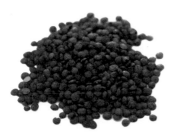

Pan-fried fillet of spicy cod on braised Puy lentils and endive salad, with a spicy tomato dressing

(serves 4)

1 onion, chopped

1 clove of garlic, chopped

225g Puy lentils

700ml fish stock

1 tbsp sherry vinegar

A little flour for dusting

4 x 225g fillets of cod, skinless (or substitute pollack – a more sustainable fish)

A little olive oil

For the dressing:

50ml white wine vinegar

3–4 tbsp tomato ketchup

150ml extra virgin olive oil

A dash of Tabasco

1–2 tbsp Worcester sauce

2 shallots, finely diced

2 plum tomatoes, deseeded and diced

1 tbsp basil, chopped

1 tbsp tarragon, chopped

Endive lettuce leaves, to serve, dressed with a little olive oil and balsamic vinegar

First, make the dressing. Whisk together the vinegar and ketchup, then whisk in the olive oil, Tabasco and Worcester sauce. Stir in the chopped shallots, diced tomato, basil and tarragon and set the mixture to one side. Pre-heat the oven to 180ºC / gas mark 4.

Heat a little olive oil in a pan, add the onions and garlic and sweat them gently together; do not let them burn. Add the Puy lentils and the fish stock, and simmer them for about 30 minutes. When the lentils are soft, remove the pan from the heat, drain them of any remaining liquid and stir in the sherry vinegar. Lightly flour the cod. Put a little olive oil in a frying pan over a high heat, and when it is hot quickly sear the fish until golden. Transfer the cod fillets to an ovenproof dish and place them in the oven for about 5 minutes.

Put a spoonful of the lentils on the centre of each plate and put some dressed endive lettuce leaves on top. When the fish is ready, place it on top of the endive and spoon the dressing around.

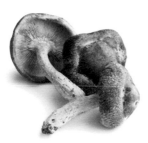

Fillet of beef with Thai green risotto and shiitake mushrooms

(serves 4)

4 120g organic fillet steaks

2 tbsp light soy sauce

2 tbsp rice wine

2 tbsp sugar

3 garlic cloves, crushed

3 tsp ground coriander

1 tsp ground ginger

1 tsp cornflour

50g fresh shiitake mushrooms

1 tbsp thick soy sauce

4 sprigs chervil

For the risotto:

4 shallots, finely chopped

750 ml vegetable stock

100g Arborio rice

finely grated zest and juice of 3 limes

2 tsp Thai green curry paste

4 lime leaves

½ tsp fresh ginger, grated

3 tbsp fromage frais

2 tbsp coconut milk

Salt

1 bunch coriander, chopped

1 bunch basil, chopped

Cut each steak horizontally into three thin medallions, then lightly beat each medallion until it is about 2 mm thick. Mix the light soy sauce, rice wine, sugar, garlic, coriander, ginger and cornflour together, then brush the mixture over the medallions and place in the fridge for 2 hours to marinate.

To make the risotto, dry-sweat the shallots in a thick-bottomed saucepan over a low heat – do not let them colour. Meanwhile, heat the stock. Add the rice to the shallots, together with the lime zest, curry paste and lime leaves; stir well. Add the stock a ladleful at a time, stirring frequently so that the starch is released. Add the stock gradually; bring to the boil and let the rice absorb the liquid before adding more. This will take 15–20 minutes. When the rice is swollen and all the stock has been used, remove the lime leaves and stir in ginger, lime juice, fromage frais and coconut milk. Season to taste with a little salt and then stir in the chopped coriander and basil. Put to one side and keep warm.

Steam the shiitake mushrooms for 5 minutes, heat a non-stick pan over a high heat and cook the beef for 1 ½ minutes on each side. Finish cooking the mushrooms in the pan in which you have cooked the beef.

To serve, place the risotto on a plate and layer the beef and mushrooms on top of it. Drizzle with thick soy sauce and garnish with chervil.

> Shiitake mushrooms stimulate the immune system to produce more interferon, which can fight off viral attack and combat cancer. Shiitake contains another active compound, eritadenine, which has been shown to lower cholesterol.

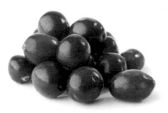

Puddings

Spiced apple, pear and cranberry crumble
(serves 6)
450g Bramley apples
450g pears
100g fresh cranberries
50g muscovado sugar
½ tsp ground cinnamon
4 tbsp rum
Zest and juice of 1 orange
4 tbsp water

For the crumble:
175g low-fat spread
200g wholemeal flour
125g porridge oats
25g flaked hazelnuts
25g demerara sugar
50g chopped dried mixed fruit
   (a mixture of apricot, cranberry and date)

Pre-heat the oven to 190ºC / gas mark 5. Peel, core and then slice the apples and the pears into chunky wedges and put them into a saucepan with the cranberries, muscovado sugar, cinnamon, rum, the orange juice and 4 tbsp of water. Cook gently, until the apples and pears are just tender. Spoon the mixture into a shallow ovenproof dish, big enough to fill to a depth of about 2.5cm, and deep enough to allow room for the crumble to go on top.

Now make the crumble. In a mixing bowl, rub the low-fat spread into the flour and oats until the crumble mixture resembles breadcrumbs. Stir in the hazelnuts, demerara sugar, dried fruit and the zest of the orange. Then scatter this evenly over the apple mixture. Bake for 25–30 minutes, until golden. Serve with low-fat crème fraiche.

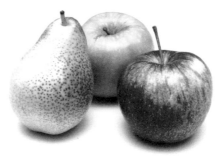

Oatmeal muesli bars

(makes about 10 bars)
200g wholemeal flour
300g porridge oats
225g dried red berries (or other dried fruit)
100g sunflower and pumpkin seeds, mixed
Zest of half an orange
Zest of half a lemon
1 tsp baking powder
175g demerara sugar
200ml rapeseed oil
125ml semi-skimmed milk
2 tbsp wild flower honey

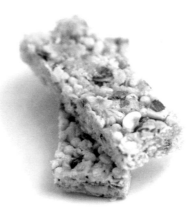

You will need a baking tin about 20 x 15 cm in size, lined with baking paper. Pre-heat the oven to 150ºC / gas mark 2. Place the flour, oats, dried berries or fruit, seeds, the orange and lemon zests and baking powder in a large mixing bowl and stir them all together. Over a low heat, and using a non-stick pan, warm the sugar, oil, milk and honey. When all the sugar has dissolved, pour this onto the oat mix and stir again, until everything is well combined. Pour the mix into the baking tray and spread it out evenly. Put it in the oven and cook it for 15–20 minutes; check to make sure it's not burning. Remove the baking tray from the oven and mark the mix into ten portions with a knife, but do not cut through to the bottom. Allow it to cool in the tin. Once cool, turn onto a wire rack and break into the marked bars. Eat the bars cold – or reheat them slightly in the microwave and serve with crème fraiche or fromage frais.

In winter, choose these seasonal foods
Pomegranate, cabbage, carrots, turnips, chicory, halibut, turkey, scallops, mussels and guinea fowl.

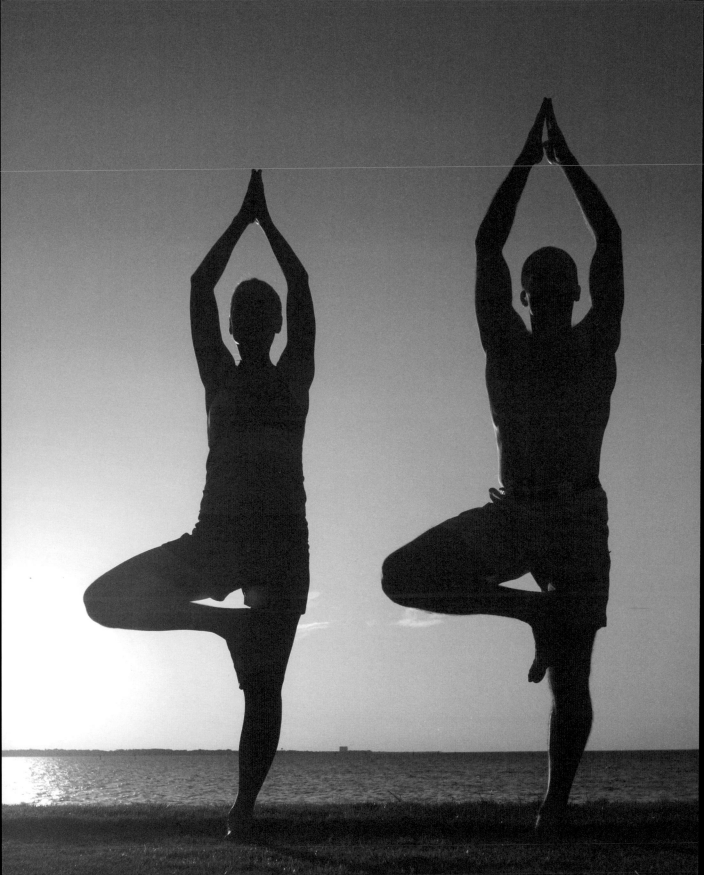

Move

Winter is a quiet, inward time – a good time to explore yoga, the ancient spiritual system of marrying movement, mind and breath. People who practise regularly nearly always cite yoga as helping them in dealing with stress and they are, almost without exception, slimmer and more youthful than their peers. Now research has given credence to the anecdotal evidence: yoga really does keep you young.

If you do not already practise yoga, below is a taster routine that will promote general well-being. You may also benefit from joining a local class that teaches yoga at the appropriate level. Try it instead of your usual stretches or any time you are feeling stressed. Spend some time learning these postures so you do not need to refer to the book. When each pose flows into the next one, you'll really feel the benefits. Come out of poses by reversing the actions so that movements are smooth, not jerky.

(Please note that these suggestions assume that you are in good general health. If you are, or could be, pregnant, or have any known health condition please consult your G.P. and a qualified yoga teacher.)

A ten-minute yoga routine

Warm up before beginning poses, and use a yoga mat or a non-slip towel to perform them on. Remember to breathe deeply and evenly through the nose. If possible take four to six breaths while holding each posture. Be calm and relaxed in the pose without strain or undue effort, only gradually extending the length of time that you hold it. Keep attentive to your breath and as you exhale feel that you surrender more deeply to the detail of the posture.

Standing

Mountain pose
Stand with the feet parallel and together if possible, a little apart if necessary for stability. Spread the toes and the balls of the feet as wide as you can and distribute the weight of the body evenly

between the balls and the heels of the feet. Think of lifting (tensing) the calf and front thigh muscles (quads) to straighten the legs rather than over-extending or locking the knees. Lift the pelvic floor muscles but keep the waist (diaphragm) relaxed. Lengthen the spine and neck, thinking of allowing the rib cage to float above the hips. Let the shoulder blades come closer together to open the upper back. The chin is slightly lowered so that the 'summit' of the Mountain is the crown of the head. Extend the arms and fingers downwards to the earth and feel that you are rising above it. Be still. Your attention is with the breath, lips together, lower jaw relaxed. Close your eyes if you wish.

Palm tree

Benefits: Stretches and tones the whole body. Swaying palm tree exercises the waist and diaphragm, releasing tensions in the respiratory system. Improves physical and mental balance.

From the Mountain pose, interlink the fingers and thumbs. Keeping your gaze on the ground a couple of metres in front, turn the palms away from you, breathe in and raise the arms above your head. Stretch as tall as you can, taking care not to over-arch the back. Think of lengthening, like a tall, willowy palm tree. After a couple of breaths in the posture, gently stretch sideways from the hips as far as comfortable on an exhalation. Hold the lateral stretch just for two or three breaths before inhaling to centre. Before releasing to the other side, change the interlock of the hands so that the other little finger is on the outside. Take care not to turn the shoulders as you stretch sideways. Remember to count your breaths and extend into the posture for the same number of breaths on each side.

Variations: Rise on to the balls of the feet. As well as trying the swaying palm tree on your toes you can also remain centred and stretch one leg forwards or backwards off the floor, balancing on the toes of one foot.

Warrior pose

Benefits: extremely good for lower back. Also extends chest and lung capacity. When it's time for action we want to remain calm and centred and face challenges with strength of mind and purpose.

Jump or step the legs as wide as comfortable. Turning the legs from the hips, rotate the left leg inwards a little and the right leg outwards about 90 degrees so that the right foot is in line with your mat. The

Five ways yoga slows down ageing

In addition to the many benefits of yoga it can help to slow down ageing.
Research studies have shown that yoga helps to:

- Maintain or lose weight along with strengthening and toning the muscles and increase flexibility.
- Ease pain – it's been shown to be particularly helpful with the relief of back pain.
- Improve sleep. Three months of practice and you should be sleeping better.
- Decrease stress. One class a week can help to reduce the stress hormone cortisol as you learn to control your mental and physical habits through the various practices of yoga, including meditation, breathing exercises and postures.
- Keep your skin elastic. Ten days of yoga can reduce the 'oxidative stress' that results in the breakdown of the skin's framework, collagen.

heel of the right foot should be roughly in line with the arch of the left foot. Leaving the legs turned to the right turn the hips and torso to the front, taking care not to twist or strain the right knee. Adjust the legs or hips if necessary. Be calm and centred, aware of the breath, as you are in Mountain pose even though the legs are in a different position. Breathing in, turn your neck, head and gaze to the right, raising both arms to shoulder height, palms down, shoulders down, arms reaching away from the shoulder blades. Breathing out, think of extending energy beyond your fingertips, looking along and beyond the right middle finger. On the next inhalation, think of lifting (tensing) the right quads in order to bend the knee until the shin is vertical and the knee is directly above the ankle. Feel that you are rising to the challenge and willing to accept it. Keep the torso centred and upright, right hip and thigh rotating outwards, left leg straight and stretching the outside of the foot into the floor. Stay in the posture for four to six breaths. When ready, inhale and straighten the right knee, head to centre, exhale and lower the arms. Repeat on the other side.

When your battles are resolved return to Mountain pose for a few quiet moments.

Lying

Spinal twist

Benefits: Opens out the chest and shoulders and releases tension in the back.

Lie on your back, knees bent, feet on the floor, hip-width apart. Take your arms out to the sides, rotating the shoulders, arms, palms upwards. Keep the arms relaxed on the floor with the hands a little lower than the shoulders. As you exhale, keep the feet on the floor just rolling hips, knees, legs and feet to the right while the neck and head roll to the left. Inhale returning to centre, then exhale to the other side. Continue the movement dynamically with the breath, releasing the bent legs to the floor each time.

Variation: For a stronger variation, hug your knees in towards your abdomen and clasp your legs under the knees, drawing them towards your chest. Feel the tension leave your hips and lower back. Relax the arms out to the sides again and continue the rolling movement as before with the breath, slowly lowering your knees to the right as you look over your left shoulder. Keep the upper back, both shoulders and arms relaxed on the floor and allow the back to do the work. Your knees and thighs should be together if possible. Flex the feet to increase the stretch. You can hold the twist for a few breaths on each side if you wish. If you are holding the posture keep both shoulders relaxed on the floor and lower the legs until they are resting comfortably on the floor. Keep your attention with the breath, releasing into the pose as you exhale, and staying for the same number of breaths each side.

Bridges

Benefits: Relieves backache. Stretches and stimulates abdominal organs and muscles and improves digestion.

Lie on your back with your arms by your sides, palms down, knees bent and your ankles below your knees, hip-distance apart. As you breathe out, contract the pelvic floor muscles, drawing the lower abdominal muscles inwards and upwards so that you tilt the pelvis and slowly peel your lower back off the floor. Now breathe in, push the feet firmly into the floor and extend the torso upwards into an arched position until only your head, neck, shoulders and feet are in contact with the floor. Take care not to distend the abdominal muscles as you lift the torso. Reach your arms along the floor towards your feet and extend the back of your neck away from your shoulders. Hold the posture for a few breaths making sure that there is no discomfort in the neck or restriction of your breath. Do not turn the neck or head while in the pose. Come down slowly on breathing out, uncurling the spine from the neck to the tail bone. Be aware of your alignment: your knees should be the same distance apart on going up and coming down.

After a couple of breaths, draw the legs up towards the chest and hold the backs of the knees. Using your arms, gently move the legs towards you and away a few times and then rock gently on the back from left to right.

Cat pose

Benefits: Restores flexibility to the spine and neck.

Start by kneeling on all fours, with your wrists below your shoulders and your knees below your hips, so that the arms and thighs are vertical and parallel. Spread the hands and fingers wide, middle fingers pointing straight forwards. Point the feet and toes so that the fronts of the ankles are stretching along the floor. The spine moves with feline grace in harmony with the breath. As you breathe out contract the pelvis and abdominal area underneath you as if you are curling your tail between your legs and extend the curve along the spine, pushing away from the floor, rounding the back like a hissing cat until your head is down and you are looking towards your tail bone. Hold the posture for a moment before breathing

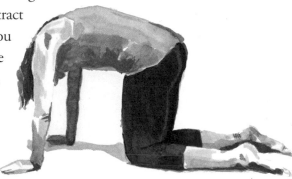

in and releasing your tail bone away, stretching into the buttocks and slowly extending the movement to arch your spine down, pulling your shoulders away from your neck. Lengthen the neck forwards lifting the head gently with a smile. Continue stretching deeply and slowly in each direction with the breath. Rest in Child's pose, below.

Child's pose

Benefits: Deeply relaxing and calming.

Sit on your heels and slowly bend forwards to rest your forehead on the floor, or on a pillow. The arms are relaxed on the floor alongside the body with the palms turned upwards and the elbows softening outwards. Relax the body and stay like this for as long as you can, feeling the breath gently in the backs of the lungs.

Downward-facing dog

Benefits: Stretches the back of the legs; reduces tension in the shoulders, stimulates the central nervous system and increases blood flow to brain and facial muscles.

Come on to your hands and knees as in the Cat pose. Curl your toes under and breathe in as you take your knees off the floor so that you are on your hands and toes. As you exhale stretch the spine backwards and upwards away from your hands, allowing your head to come towards the floor as your buttocks stretch up towards the ceiling. Focus on releasing into the shoulders as you move towards an inverted 'V' shape, with a straight back and straight legs. If possible, slowly push your heels down towards the floor and keep pressing on the heels of the hand to extend the stretch. To come out of the pose bend the knees and return to the Cat pose. Relax in Child's pose. To complete your practice, relax in the Corpse pose.

Corpse pose

Lie flat on your back in a symmetrical posture with the legs comfortably apart and the arms a little away from the body, shoulders and palms turned up. Rest the head on a pillow if more comfortable. Allow the body to be quite still as you keep your attention with the quiet flow of the breath. Let go of all control as you simply observe your body breathing.

If you wish, you can rest the legs on a chair, sofa or up against a wall. This can help to lengthen and relax the back muscles.

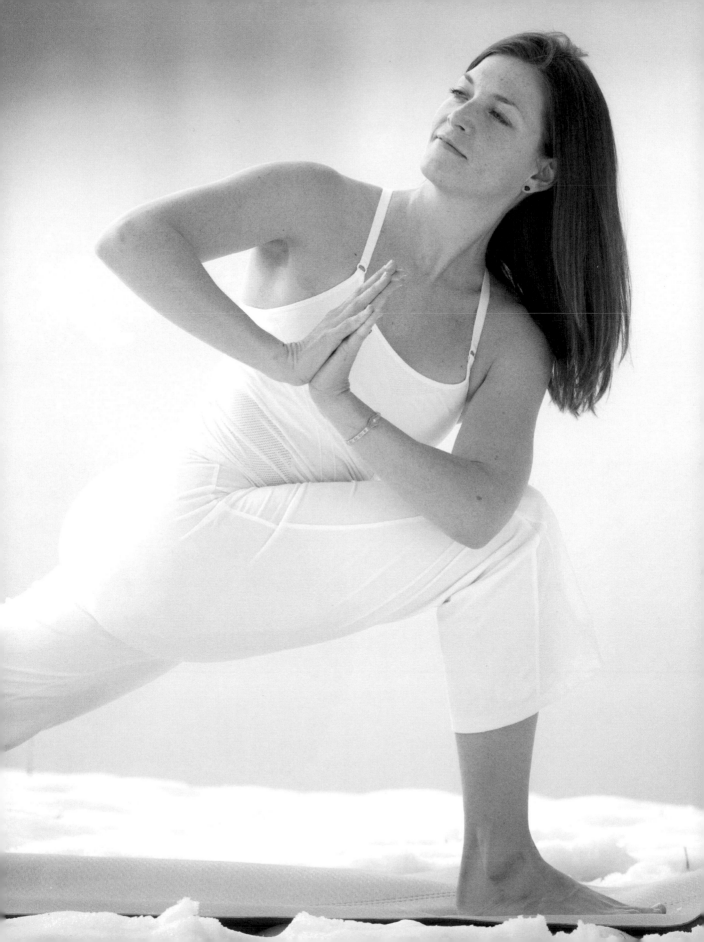

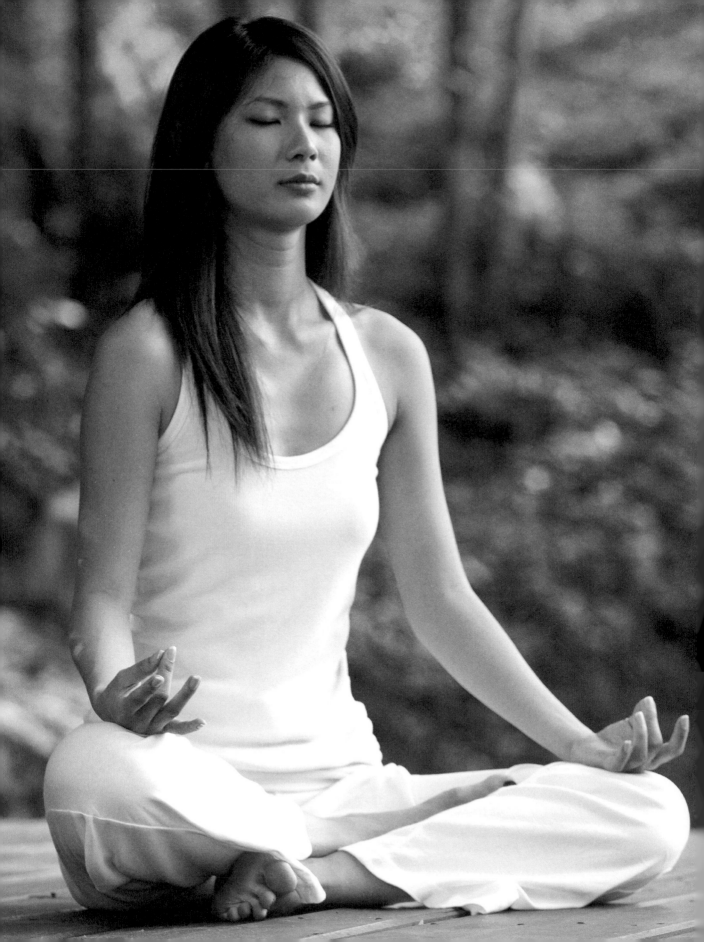

Try these traditional Eastern practices

To detox

This back-stretching pose tones and massages the entire abdominal and pelvic region including the liver, pancreas, spleen, reproductive system and adrenal glands. This increases blood flow to these areas and helps to detoxify and strengthen all the organs. It will work well with the Be Revitalised programme on page 285.

Releasing pose

Lie on your back, drawing your knees up to your chest, with one hand on each knee or behind your knees if you have knee problems. Breathe out, squeeze your thighs and knees as close to the torso and chest as possible so that the right thigh is putting pressure on the ascending colon and the left thigh on the descending colon. Breathing in, release your knees and thighs away from your torso without letting go of them.

Because this pose also stretches the lower back it stimulates the kidneys, providing an all round detoxing effect. To increase the action of the pose you can include the neck and head by bringing your head between your knees on exhalation and returning it to the floor on inhalation, taking care not to tense the shoulders. These should curl up off the floor but not lift up to your ears.

This posture should not be practised after eating (for obvious reasons) otherwise it is safe to do on its own, unless you are pregnant or have recently had abdominal surgery.

For calm

Rhythmic breathing

Deep breathing is used to help induce calm and complete relaxation in many traditional and modern exercise disciplines, while also returning you to a sense of centredness. You can practise this lying or sitting.

Either lie down with your arms relaxed beside your body or sit cross-legged on the floor or on a chair with your hands resting on your knees. Breathe through your nose with your eyes and mouth closed, dropping your lower jaw inside your mouth. Focus on your breathing, first of all feeling the breath at your nostrils and upper lip. Then concentrate your attention on your abdomen and become aware of how it inflates on the inhalation and flattens on the exhalation. Be aware of the gentle movement of your ribcage. As you exhale feel any tension or anxiety melting away while affirming this in your mind. Bring an even count to your breath, inhaling for four counts, then exhaling for four counts. If you wish you can also hold your breath for two counts – that is, breathe in for four counts, hold for two counts, breathe out for four counts and hold for two counts. To conclude the exercise, stop counting and observe the breath settle back into its own rhythm. When you are ready gently stretch the whole body and open your eyes.

Anti-ageing

The 'carrying the moon' pose is said by the Chinese to enhance youthfulness as it gives you a supple spine which is essential if you want to be alert physically and mentally. The Chinese say that 'you need not worry about growing old if your spine is young!' as the spine is the home of the nerves that run to the entire body.

'Carrying the moon'

From an ordinary upright position, slowly exhale while bending your body forwards, so your hands drop below your knees. Tuck your head in so that your whole back makes a smooth curve, pause for a few seconds and visualise the flow of vital energy going up your spine to your head. Then bring your body up, straightening your arms forwards and upwards in a continuous movement, gently breathing in until you reach the highest point. With your thumbs and index fingers forming a wide 'V' shape – as if you are holding a full moon above you – move them behind your head, so you are slightly arching your head backwards. Hold and pause for a few seconds while looking at the moon formed by your fingers. Straighten your body and lower your arms down to your sides, breathing out gently. At the same time, visualise vital energy flowing from your head downwards in all directions, as if an internal shower was swishing away all the dust, rust and negative energy into the ground.

Quicker than surgery

Use Chinese medicine to banish wrinkles and remove signs of tiredness. Here is a quick exercise using an ancient Qigong practice that you can do whenever you are tired. It will improve circulation to the face and energise it.

• Place the tip of your tongue against the roof of your mouth. Inhale deeply while rubbing your hands together for about a minute, until they feel warm.

• Press your palms against your closed eyes for ten seconds or so, exhaling and focusing on the energy and warmth penetrating your eyes.

• Rest your hands on either side of your nose and lightly massage your face outwards from the nose to the ears, imagining your skin becoming ever smoother.

• Now stroke your face, massaging it with your palms from the chin to the hairline (as you do this your two middle finger tips should touch the sides of your nose). When your finger tips reach the hairline, separate your hands and massage along the hairline, over the temples, in front of the ears and over the jaw, then returning to your chin again. Repeat this eighteen times.

The TV workout

In winter it's easy to make excuses. But there are none. You can exercise, even if you do it in front of the TV (and you can adapt this for your office, too). Here are some suggestions.

- Wall push-ups for the upper body. Stand with your feet hip-distance apart, with your palms flat against a wall, at shoulder height and shoulder-width apart. Bring your upper body slowly towards the wall, keeping navel to spine and then push yourself back to the start position. Avoid moving the feet and keep your body in a straight line from heel to head during the exercise. Repeat twelve times.

- Squats for the lower body. Before you sit down to watch the TV or begin your day at work, practise lowering and lifting your bum. Stand with your feet slightly wider than shoulder -width apart. Bend your knees, lean forwards from the hips, push your bum out behind and squat down imagining you were going to sit in your chair, but as your bum gets level with your knees, you change your mind. Rise from the squat to a standing position, keeping your chest lifted. Keep your navel in to support the lower back throughout the exercise. Repeat twelve times. See the illustration on page 117.

- Build core strength. If your job requires spending long periods of time sitting then sit on a stability ball – one of those large plastic balls – instead of a normal seat. This builds core strength by challenging balance and requires you to hold good posture.

In addition to these, all the body conditioning exercises and stretches starting on pages 117 and 123 can be performed at home while watching the TV. Give them a go. Keep up the cardio exercise during the winter months. It can improve mood and has been shown to reduce stress and help beat the winter blues. Spice it up with anything new or different – whether it's a cardio machine, fitness class or DVD you have never tried or simply being more creative with the speed, intensity or duration of your chosen workout. Even the smallest changes can help you develop new enthusiasm and motivation for your workout.

Your anti-ageing priorities

Although we all aspire to optimal health and fitness, one factor that we must accept as an inevitable course of nature is the ageing process. However, ageing can be slowed down by engaging in exercise. From an anti-ageing perspective, the real question is not whether to exercise, but more importantly, what kind of exercise, how much, and how often. Anti-ageing exercises should consist of three fitness components: flexibility, cardiovascular exercise and muscular strength and endurance training. Exercise programmes must be customised to meet your personal needs, based on your current physical condition. Doing the right balance of the three activities for your age group could lead to a healthier life and a slowing of the ageing process.

In your twenties or thirties:

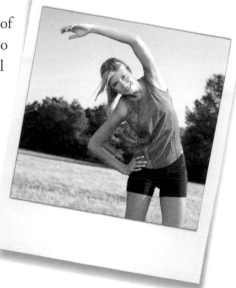

• Priority: your main aim is to build a strong foundation of fitness to help your anti-ageing battle in later life. Cardio activities will boost energy levels and resistance training will target your muscle strength and tone. Specifically, women in their child-bearing years also benefit from postural exercises as well as core-stabilisation and pelvic floor exercises - all essential for later years in life.

• Don't think 'I'm so young I don't have to bother'. Furring of your arteries and osteoporosis can start by the time you are out of your teens.

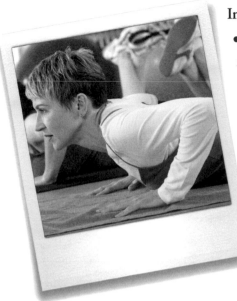

In your forties:

• Priority: you need to focus on resistance training to keep your metabolism revved up and build the strength to replace lost muscle. Aim to be physically active every day.

• Don't make the mistake of being lulled into a false sense of security by thinking that because your brain is busy, your body is, too. Rushing around does not translate into physical fitness.

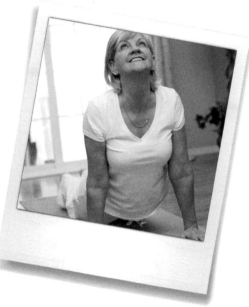

In your fifties:

• Priority: prevent middle-aged spread. Work on perfecting your abdominal and back-strengthening exercises, in particular you need to master the navel to spine connection to help keep your midriff toned.

• Don't forget that this is a decade of mood swings and big changes. Cardiovascular exercise is a superb mood regulator and stress buster. Do some form of it every day.

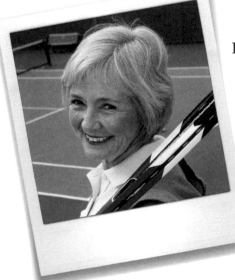

In your sixties or more:

• Priority: maintaining strength and flexibility. Take regular walks and swims, and stretch.

• Don't think 'it's too late'. Studies have shown that people into their seventies and eighties have experienced positive benefits from regular exercise.

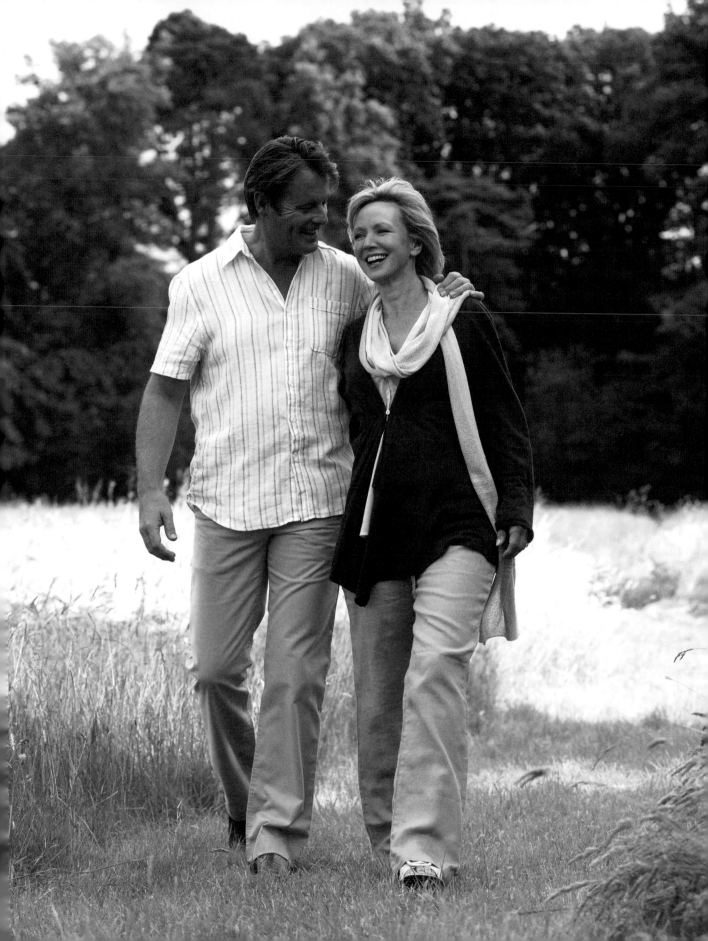

Deep comfort, treatments as relaxing as a hot bath after a long day or a cold night. Sink into these.

Love yourself

Spa Heaven Cocoon

This is the ultimate body treatment including an exfoliation, warm body wrap, and a head and foot massage. Indulgent oriental spa recipes will leave your skin feeling smooth and silky and looking luminous, and the foot and head massage will result in a deeply relaxed state of mind.

Champneys Oriental Sensual Body Mist, Champneys Oriental Body Glow and Champneys Oriental Body Cream are strongly recommended; this treatment was designed around them. Otherwise use a scrub and cream that seem both indulgent and relaxing to you. You will also need a massage oil such as Champneys Pure Relaxation Massage Oil or make your own. At Champneys, this treatment uses heat to relax the muscles, and a heated blanket will really add to the experience. You will also need a clean linen double sheet and a heavy blanket, a pair of warm cotton socks and a couple of heated towels.

Before you start: Place the heated blanket – with the sheet over it – on a bed or a lounger, and switch it on. Place the heavy blanket nearby. (Do not forget to switch off the blanket before you lie down.) Mix the scrub in a bowl with your chosen massage oil. In another bowl, mix the body cream with the massage oil.

Exfoliate
In the shower or bath, apply the scrub and oil mixture. With large circles and firm strokes, work on the arms and legs, including the top of your feet. Then move to your stomach, bust and back. Shower off the scrub (preferably with Champneys Oriental Shower Cream) and wrap yourself in a heated robe or towel, then move to a warm room.

Massage
Using some of the body cream and oil mix, or a specialised foot treatment such as Champneys Intensive Cracked Heel Treatment Balm, sit on the edge of the bed and massage first the left, then the right foot (see page 141). After the massage, wear the warm cotton socks.

Using some of your chosen massage oil, warm it in your palms and apply it to your scalp with the finger tips, as if shampooing your whole head. Start at the hairline and move towards the ears and then round the back of the head. Then make small static circles, release the pressure and work your way towards the crown, leaving an inch between each movement.

With both thumbs on your earlobes, massage in circular movements to the top of the ear and back down, squeezing and pulling the lobe down. Using the palm of the hand, rotate the scalp using large circles from the hairline towards the ears and then around the back of the head. Rake your fingers through your hair from left to right three times: first time, firmly; second time, with medium pressure; third time, lightly. Gently tug your hair to finish and wrap it in the heated towel.

Now massage the whole body starting with the back, then the legs, arms and chest, with the cream and oil mixture. Move with firm long strokes.

Relax

Switch off the electric blanket – the sheet should be toasty. Wrap yourself in it and place the heavy blanket over it. Lie back and relax in your cocoon; the heat will help your skin absorb the oils. Afterwards, if possible, go straight to bed and sleep.

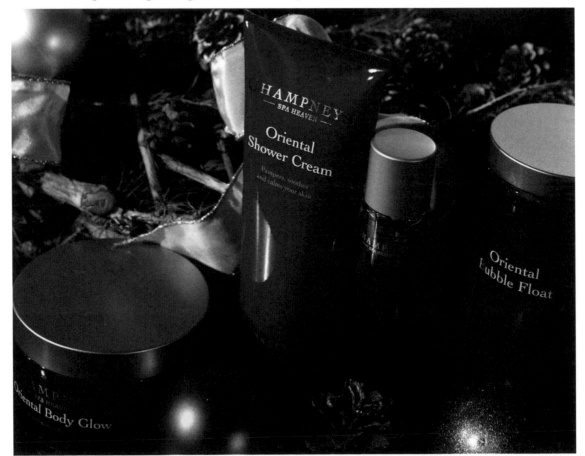

The half-hour face lift

Jo Parker, Champneys Spa Director, recommends a professional brow shape in winter (or, indeed, at any time of year). 'This opens up your eyes, giving definition to your face – some people call it the quickest, cheapest face lift. Once you have had a professional brow shape, it's easy to keep the shape by plucking out the odd stray hair yourself.'

If you do decide to shape at home, don't overdo it. Here are Jo's tips:

- Take a pencil and looking in a mirror, hold the pencil vertically with the base of the pencil touching the nostril, the top of the pencil should be lined up with the inner corner of the eye. Any hairs in the middle section of the bridge of the nose should be removed.

- Next, place the base of the pencil against the nostril – using the base of the pencil as the pivot point, slide the pencil until it reaches the outer corner of the eye (do not go lower) then remove any hairs beyond this point. As you age the eyebrow should become shorter. To create the illusion of a lifted, more open appearance, the pivot point remains the same but this time raise the pencil to the edge of the colour of your eye whilst ensuring you are looking directly forward.

- Apply a hot flannel to your brows before you start; it will make hair extraction easier.

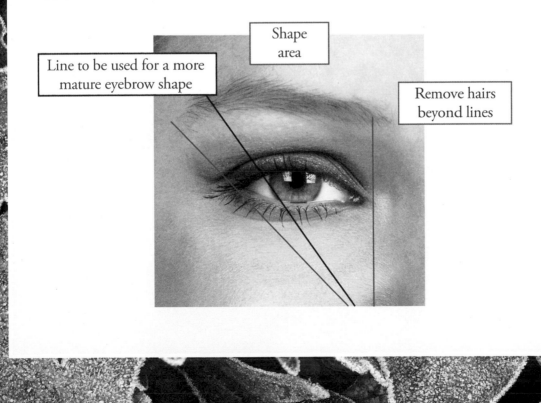

Shape area

Line to be used for a more mature eyebrow shape

Remove hairs beyond lines

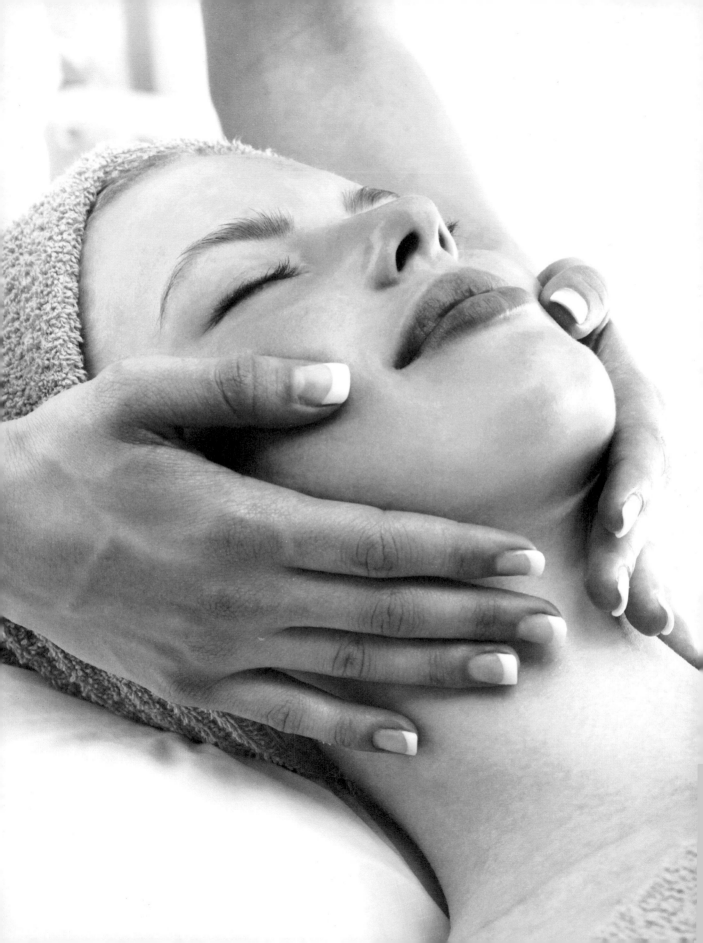

Collagen Enriched Anti-Ageing Facial

This is Champneys' hardest-working facial ever – the ultimate skin-plumping experience for those who want to prevent and smooth away the signs of ageing. It combines a traditional French method of deep brush cleansing and gentle steaming mist with Marine Collagen eye and face masks. After this treatment you should see visible results; your skin will be clean, firm, smooth and glowing.

You will need: Champneys Fresh Face Micro-Dermabrasion System with brush attachment; alternatively, a large bowl to be filled with boiling water and a complexion brush. This treatment uses Champneys Radiant Skin Double Enzyme Mask, an exfoliating mask, and Champneys Collagen Plus Range. You will need these for best results or, at the least, an eye and face mask designed to be anti-ageing.

Before you start: Prepare the Facial Steamer or pour boiling water into the large bowl.

Cleanse, exfoliate and steam

Cleanse your face thoroughly, using your normal cleanser. Tone.

Exfoliate with Champneys Fresh Face Micro-Dermabrasion System or a complexion brush following the brush routine on page 144.

Apply an exfoliating or brightening mask such as Champneys Radiant Skin Double Enzyme Mask and Collagen Enriched Anti-Ageing Eye Masks. Position the steamer or bowl at least twelve inches from your face and steam for between five and ten minutes. Remove mask(s). Tone.

Massage

Massage with Champneys Super Rich Floral Facial Balm or a few drops of oil with a couple of drops of geranium essential oil added – using Champneys' facial massage routine. This routine helps smooth out lines and release tension in the face. Once mastered, it can be used to apply moisturiser or oil whenever needed.

• Apply balm or facial oil over the face and décolletage.

• Sweep with your palms from the base of the chest bone out to the opposite shoulders, down to the elbows and back up, around the back of shoulders to the base of the skull – six times.

• Using knuckles, repeat the movement above three times.

• Vibrate with the palms of hands across the same area, three times.

• Make circular movements across the same area, three times.

• Now do sweeping movements across the same area once.

• Using alternating palms, sweep across the décolletage from one shoulder to the other. Do this once.

• Now the 'prayer' movement. The hands come to a praying position on the chin and then sweep up over the cheeks, fingers up the sides of the nose so that your hands are spread on your forehead. Do this three times.

• Use thumbs and fingers to 'wring' along the jawline from the chin to the left ear and then back, and from the chin to the right ear and then back – three times.

• Use your palms to create small vibrations on your cheeks, working from the chin outwards to the ears, three times.

• Gently knuckle your cheeks simultaneously, using upward movements, three times.

• Use firm knuckle strokes over your cheeks, from the chin up towards the ears – three times.

• Circle the nose. Use your middle fingers to circle the tip of your nose, sweep down and press at the sides of the nostrils. Circle the middle of the nose and sweep down and press at the side of the nose. Circle the top of the nose and sweep up to press in the middle of the eyebrows. Do this three times.

• Use the middle three fingers to circle your eyes, moving out over the top of the eyes and in underneath them, six times.

• Drain and circle your eyes using index and middle fingers to press out over the eyebrows, pinching the eyebrows between the fingers. Repeat, using your middle fingers to create small circles and work back underneath the eyes to the nose. Press at the middle of the eyebrows, six times.

• Use the middle three fingers to create small circular movements over your forehead, lifting upwards towards the hairline. Start in the centre of your forehead just above the eyebrows and work out towards the ears. Sweep back to the centre and repeat this over the entire forehead.

• Palm squeeze. Sweep your hands around so the heels of the hands are on your temples and your fingers are interlocked. Squeeze your temples and pull in an upwards direction. Release the squeeze and repeat three times.

Afterwards…

Apply Champneys Collagen Plus Anti-Wrinkle Eye Treatment – or an equivalent – with the 'Zorro' application. You do this by using only the index and middle fingers. Press the centre of your eyebrows with the index fingers six times. Sweep with four fingers from the inner corners of the eye to the temples like a mask, and do so three times. Circle at the temples three times.

Apply Champneys Super Calm Lip Balm with your ring finger around your lips. Apply Champneys Collagen Enriched Anti-Ageing Face Mask, or a similar mask, over your face, neck and décolletage. Place damp cotton wool pads on your eyes and relax for the time specified on the pack.

Remove the masks, then apply eye gel using the 'Zorro' application and moisturise using Champneys Collagen Plus or your usual moisturiser.

Optional finish: apply a product designed to give radiance, such as Champneys Perfect Skin Illuminating Beauty Balm.

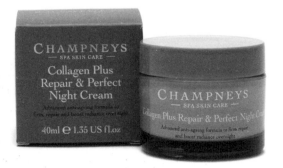

'Exfoliation is my number one tip. Getting rid of dead cells makes skin glow.'

– JO PARKER, CHAMPNEYS' SPA DIRECTOR AND BEAUTY EXPERT

Hot Stone Therapy

Why massaging with hot stones is quite so relaxing but invigorating, too, is something of a mystery – but it definitely works. Obviously, nothing can beat a professionally trained therapist for the complete experience of a hot stone massage, but you can still tap into the power of the stones in your own home. Next time you're strolling on a beach look for smooth stones about as big as a woman's palm or a little smaller.

Clean them thoroughly and then place them in a bowl of boiling water and leave them to heat up. Remove them with tongs and put them on a towel until they have cooled sufficiently to place on your skin without any risk of burning. Work quickly when they are cool enough to use, as they lose heat fast.

Some ideas:

- Ask a partner or a friend to place them on your back, running along the curve of the shoulder blades in the middle of the back and then running down either side of your spine.

- Use a larger stone to massage the soles of your feet.

- Run a larger stone across your shoulders to help relieve tension.

- Lie a larger than usual stone on the small of your back.

- Place some smaller stones across the top of your eyebrows and place one on your 'third eye'.

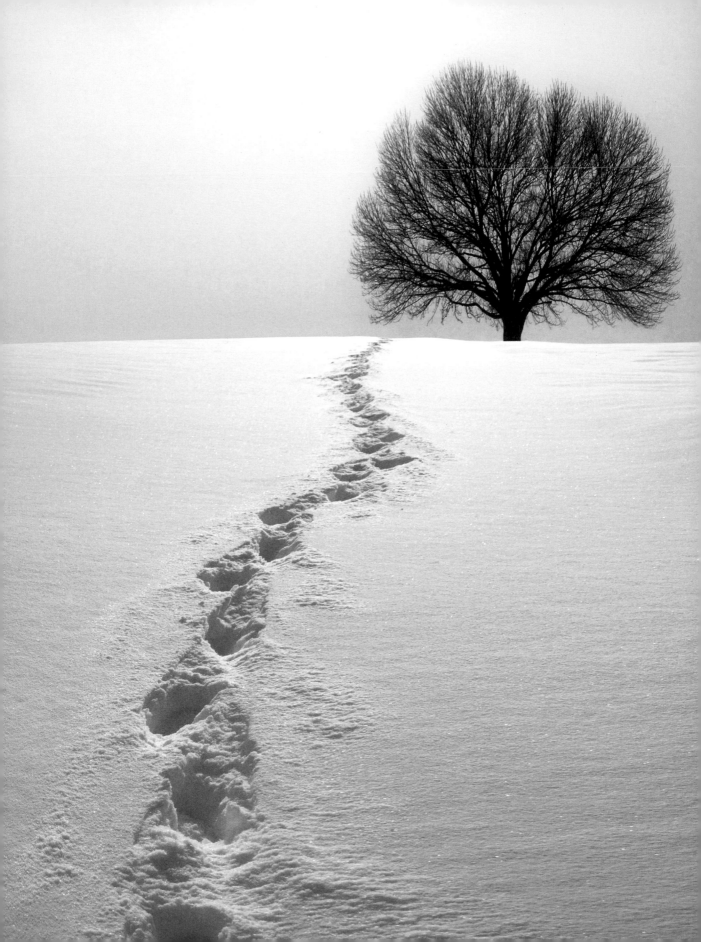

Well-being

Finding your path home...

In mid-winter we often make a journey home, a journey back to where we come from. But it's also traditionally a time which lends itself to a spiritual journey inwards, when we can determine if our life is still on course. It is a time for insights and 'aha' moments, self-examination, self-knowledge and self-discovery.

This is the time for asking if you are happy in your skin, happy with the person you are turning into, happy with the life choices you've made already. It's time to dig deep and become reacquainted with yourself so that, come spring, you'll be ready to meet new challenges and make changes if changes have to be made.

Below are some ideas to begin this project of self-exploration. Switch off the TV, light a candle and feel a thrill of excitement at what you might achieve next year. These exercises make perfect material for contemplation on long evenings in front of the fire.

Remember your 'starring' roles?

We are all given the chance to be 'stars'. We are given the opportunity to have a huge impact on other people's lives but sometimes we forget that to certain key people we really matter. Often a hectic life means we just lose sight of it. When you're feeling that you're doing a lot but not doing any of it properly, working out if you are playing a bit part in a not very important movie to the detriment of the starring role you could have elsewhere is a worthwhile reminder of what's important in life. Try this:

• Think what roles you fulfil in life. The list might look like this: 'wife, mother, daughter, accountant, sister, charity worker, PTA member, friend'.

• Now rewrite your list but put them in order not of who is most important but who is really getting most of your time. Now the list might look like: 'accountant, mother, friend, wife, charity worker, sister, daughter, PTA member'.

• Finally, place the roles in the order of importance in your life.

This in itself can be a reminder of how life can get out of kilter, with the most important people getting too little attention, but it can also be a help in prioritising time. Next time you are in a dilemma as to whether you should keep your boss happy and work late, or make your sister happy and arrive at her birthday party on time, your list will remind you that 'sister' is much more important than 'employee', but that she won't know it unless – most of the time – you behave as if she is.

Rediscover your creativity

We're all inherently creative, but by about the age of seven most of us have begun to put that side of ourselves in a box marked 'not for me'. This winter, rediscover that creative side. It can prove absorbing, relaxing and stimulating. It can help you think laterally and view the world in a different way.

At first you don't have to be formal. Think about some art or craft you've always been interested in and set aside an hour a week to pursue it. Research on the Internet by all means, but don't spend your time reading how to do it – actually start. It doesn't have to be good, it just has to be interesting and absorbing. You don't have to start with oil painting, you can buy a child's colouring book and some crayons and lose yourself in creating a world where you get to decide on everything. Stick with this journey and you'll be amazed at where it can take you.

'I'm always doing things I can't do. That's how I get to do them.'
– PABLO PICASSO

An easy meditation

Meditation gives peace of mind, relief from stress, brilliant ideas, better health and an enviable lightness of spirit. But we think of it as something hard and daunting. Instead, switch your mindset. All we're suggesting is that you simply 'be'. Simply be still for a few moments a day…

- Sit in any comfortable position – in a chair, cross-legged on a meditation cushion or on the floor. Relax your jaw and breathe regularly. Close your eyes. Relax each group of muscles in turn.

- Inhale through your nose.

- Exhale through your nose and say inwardly any word that calms you – 'peace', 'om', 'love', 'holiday'.

- Repeat. When your mind wanders – and it will – observe your thoughts, then let them go and bring your focus back to your power word.

- Gently come out of your meditation. Stretch.

Any time spent meditating is good. Start with just a few minutes and build up. Even ten minutes a day can have a profoundly relaxing effect on your life.

Reconnect with those you love

Intimacy means sharing experiences, feelings and thoughts. It means wanting to hang out with your partner more than with just about anyone else. But in even the best relationships this intimacy can dwindle as the demands of family and work encroach into your time and energy. The early months of the year, culminating in Valentine's Day, are a quiet time and a natural space in the calendar to focus on your closest personal relationships. How do you get the intimacy back? Here is a starter.

John Gottman, who has researched the differences between happy and unhappy couples in detail, has identified four dynamics that can wreck a relationship: being critical, defensiveness, stonewalling and contempt. It seems obvious, but it's extraordinary how easy it is to fall into these dynamics when a conflict arises. Treating your partner respectfully and not saying unkind things just to be right goes a long way to resolving arguments. Gottman discovered that couples who routinely resolve problems, and grow stronger as a result, say on average five positive statements for every single negative one. This is a good discipline to put in place when you are having problems. Speaking positively in a ratio of five to one makes it much harder to fall into relationship-wrecking behaviours.

Unrecognised emotions are often at the root of lack of intimacy. The most common is fear – fear of rejection, fear of illness, pain or of being alone. The fear can manifest itself in either partner (or both) as anger, indifference, workaholism, depression, drinking too much or another form of 'absenteeism' from the relationship, like throwing yourself into caring for the children. Spending time working out how you really feel about your life and your loved ones and expressing that to them (yes, you need to talk) can help bring these emotions out into the open quickly. Meditation can help with self awareness (see page 279.)

Finally, play with your partner. Remember the five to one ratio again – five positive experiences for every negative one. Book time out every week to have fun together. Every month try something new as a couple – a new sport, an entertainment, a weekend break. (Have you visited a spa together? Shedding stress in a few hours can work wonders for your relationship.)

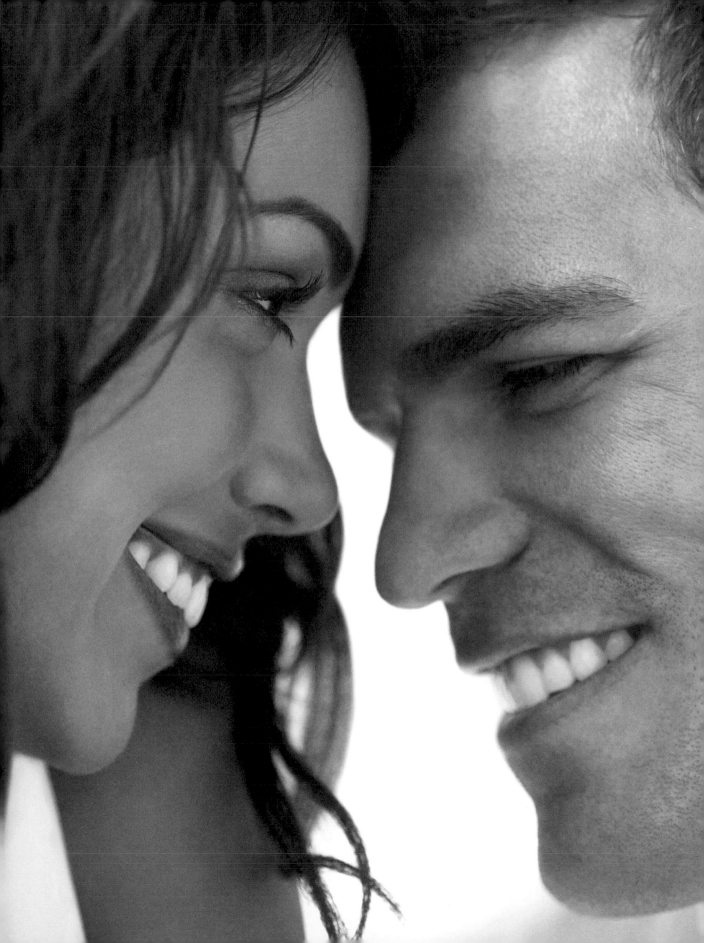

Reconnect with what makes you happy

Recognising what you really love means that you can start bringing more of it into your life, which should make you more content. Or you can use this exercise as the springboard for planning a completely new working life based on what really makes your heart sing.

When do you lose yourself?
Think back to the last time you were so completely engrossed in what you were doing that you didn't notice time passing. Were you painting a room, listening to your friend talk, dancing at a wedding, decorating a cake? Were you driving, shopping, helping with homework? What do you commit to, even when you are frantically busy – the PTA, the book club, your monthly facial? Write it down. Remember what you loved as a child. Were you happier on your own or with other people, in the garden or at the swimming pool? Study your list. Mull on what you've come up with. Imagine ways you could be in that atmosphere much more of the time.

What do you dream about?
If you won the lottery, what would you spend your time doing for love rather than money? Any clues there?

What are you afraid of?
What's stopping you fulfilling your dreams? Are you afraid to tell your partner? Or to give up a lucrative job that bores you? The longer you've worked in a profession, the harder it is to walk away from it – but thinking of a career change as transferring skills rather than starting again can help. There are not always easy solutions to finding time to pursue your passions, but recognising what is stopping you is a first step in realising those dreams. Once recognised, problems have a way of transforming and melting away.

Where are the soulmates?
Go back to your first question. Include more of what makes you happy in your life and you'll meet people who share your interests. Who knows what richness they will add to your life or where it will take you?

Reclaim the night

Surveys show that we are all working longer hours than ever before if domestic chores are added into the equation (around thirteen hours a day!). Reclaim your evenings as chill-out time. Choose a time that makes sense (sometime between 7–8 p.m., say) and promise yourself that you won't do any work, of any kind, when you reach that watershed. Mark the beginning of your evening proper with a 'transition ritual' – a shower, bath, meditation or simply a change into comfortable clothes. 'Passive relaxation' (basically, the TV) is not as relaxing as 'active relaxation'. This is what active relaxation looks like…

- A few yoga stretches.
- One of the Champneys spa treatments.
- A walk or swim.
- Popping to the local pool for a sauna or steam.
- Reading or listening to music.

Downing tools also makes it easier to find the time to reconnect with friends on the phone or Internet. Maintaining what's called 'social contact' and a healthy network of family and friends is a proven way to keep young.

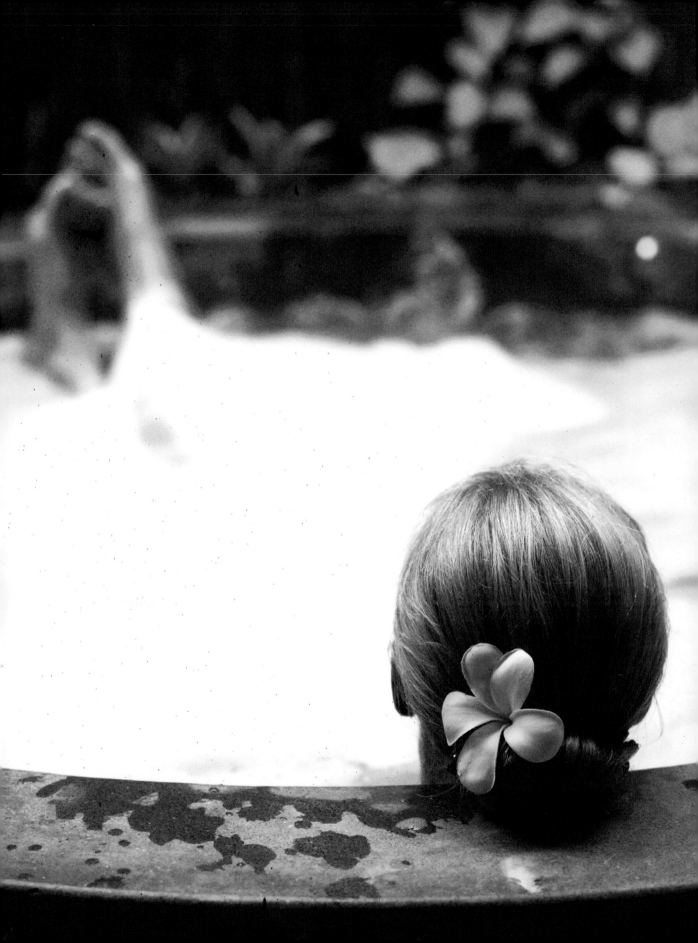

Escape – Be revitalised

Winter is a season of extremes – it's a time for going inwards and connecting with our deeper selves. But we also party harder in winter than any other time of the year. No wonder we sometimes feel overwhelmed, confused and just plain exhausted and that's probably why winter is always a busy time at Champneys. Prior to Christmas, guests arrive for some rest and relaxation before the party season begins. After Christmas, they come to recover.

A spa break appeals because our guests want a break from exhaustion, other people's demands, heavy food and too much booze. A few days of making themselves the priority – and some delicious but healthy food – restores them and helps them maintain their weight, too.

If you can't book yourself into a Champneys' Resort this winter, here is the next best thing: a short programme that will have you relaxed and raring to go even in the midst of winter. It serves as a 'mini detox' – you should lose a few pounds – but the main purpose of the revitalising programme is to restore your energy levels, shake off fatigue and bring back your joie de vivre – very fast indeed.

The programme mimics the sort of five-day stay you would have at a Champneys Resort. OK, it won't be quite as relaxing, but it is amazing what you can achieve with some determination to prioritise yourself. Remember that you won't have the energy to give to other people if you don't nurture yourself.

The Champneys 'little black dress' regime
– your five-day revitalising programme

The programme is the same every day, but what is important is that you make a serious plan and stick to it. Draw a grid for the five days you are going to follow the programme and under each day plan exactly what you are going to eat, when you are going to exercise and what treatments you are going to schedule in. Then make sure you have bought everything you need; it is essential to be organised. This is also a low-calorie regime, so shouldn't be followed for more than five days – otherwise your body may go into 'starvation' mode which will mean that when you do start to eat properly, you'll feel worse and weigh more than you did before.

These rules apply for each day:

- Eat five times a day – three meals and two snacks.

- Drink two litres of water and/or green tea every day.

- Exercise every day.

- Don't eat carbohydrates (with the exception of vegetables) after 5 p.m.

- Limit carbohydrates to good-quality wholegrains and have no more than two portions a day with breakfast and lunch.

- Ground yourself and dissipate stress with a body-pampering treat every day.

- Be in bed by 11 p.m. at the latest – earlier if possible.

What to eat

- Concentrate on eating lean protein and vegetables. Cutting down on carbohydrate will help you lose any excess water and thus cut down on bloating. It isn't 'real' weight loss, but it will make you feel better in that little black dress.

- Eat a breakfast and lunch which consist of a small portion (three tablespoons) of good-quality carbs, like wholemeal pasta or brown rice, and an equal amount of lean protein. Your choices could be rice with tuna, a thin slice of wholegrain bread with an egg, pasta and chicken. Fill up with vegetables.

- Mid-morning and mid-afternoon, snack on fruit or fruit juice. Have a handful of nuts twice a day with the fruit, to fill you up for longer.

- For dinner have vegetables and protein. (Embrace protein on this programme. It will give you the energy to avoid hunger and bingeing.)

- Avoid bread, biscuits, pasta, potatoes and rice except for those carbs specified above. We all need carbohydrates to feel happy and for vital energy, and cutting them out for even a short time is self-defeating, but for five days you can manage on a small amount of good-quality carb.

- Avoid dairy and substitute calcium-enriched soya products instead. At Champneys we're against cutting out any food group but, for five days, soya alone will provide the nutrients you need.

- Avoid alcohol. It's nutritionally empty and you'll have plenty of it at other times this season.

What to do

- Walk or do other cardiovascular exercise for forty minutes minimum a day.

- Do core strength exercises on the first, third and fifth day.

- Do flexibility exercises on the second and fourth day.

Exercise makes you body aware – it helps your posture and confidence. If you don't normally exercise regularly, you will actually see results in the mirror; in just a few days you can look more svelte. And if you do exercise regularly, this is the time of year when your usual commitment to exercise probably goes out the window. At least for these five days, find time for yourself.

Treat your body every day to some luxurious pampering – if you don't have time for a full treatment (but make sure you have time for some!), then promise yourself a long soak or an invigorating shower. This is a good time to book yourself in for a professional facial or toning treatment.

Give yourself one of the treatments in this book every day if you can, but at times when it's too busy at least enjoy an aromatherapy soak, body brushing, a foot bath, a body massage with oils or a face mask. Best of all, if at all possible – slip between the sheets mid-afternoon and have a lovely nap. That's what winter afternoons are for.

'Start each morning with a big 1½ litre bottle of water on your desk or workspace. Aim to drink a small glass every hour on the hour so you've emptied it by the end of the day. If you don't like the taste of plain water, add a few slices of lemon and some chunks of ginger to add flavour.'

– AILSA HIGGINS, CHAMPNEYS' NUTRITIONIST

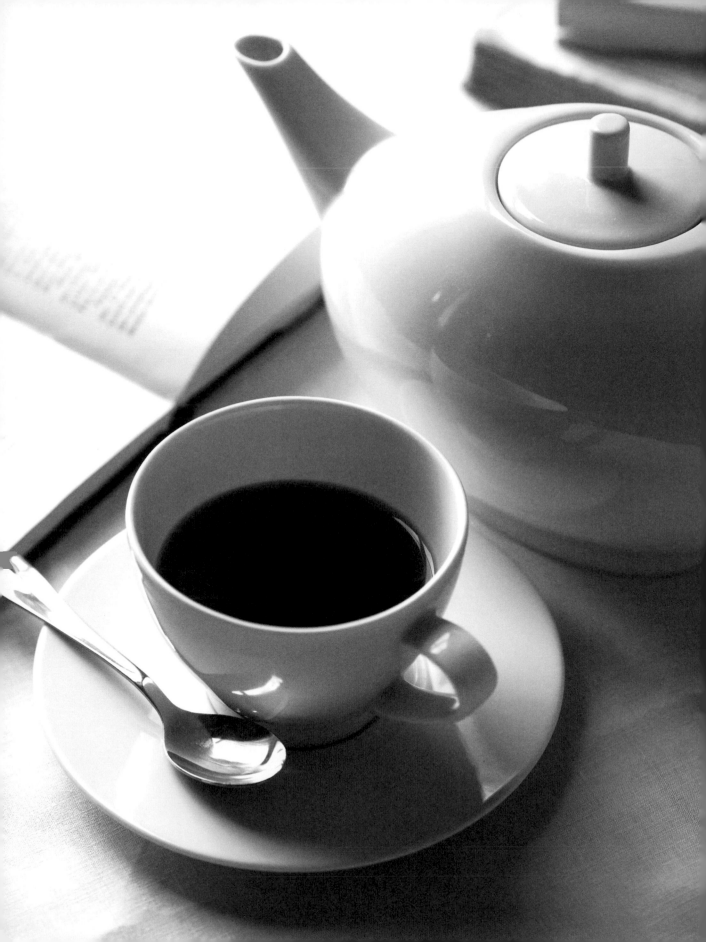

Index

A

abdominal curls 118–119
 better back programme, 196
 Pilates, 189
active relaxation, 7, 283
'adding in' healthy foods, 19, 20–22
afternoon naps, 154, 206, 267
alcohol
 'little black dress' regime, 286
 'mindful' intake, 22
Alexander Technique, 78
almond butter, 233
anorexics, micronutrient requirements, 229
anti-ageing
 Carrying the moon pose, 260
 diet, 227–236
 exercise, 251, 253, 260, 263–264
 facial, 271–273
 social contact, 283
 yoga, 251, 253
antioxidants
 anti-ageing diet, 227, 231, 232, 233, 236
 fruit, 26
 ORAC scale, 236, 239
 parsnips, 241
 pomegranates, 240
aromatherapy oils, 2–3
 anti-cellulite, 137
 detox, 66
arrow exercise (Pilates), 187
at-home spa, *see* spa treatments and pampering
autumn, 155–157
 aromatherapy oils, 3, 154
 celebrating, 154

escape, 217–219
exercise, 185–197
nutrition, 159–183
recipes, 169–182
spa treatments and pampering, 199–209
well-being, 211–214

B

back
 back care programme, 193–197
 extensions, 119, 196
 pain, 193–197, 253
 stretch, 124
back of the thigh stretch, 124
backs of upper arms stretch, 123
bananas, 24, 169
barley, 164
Be Active programme, 126, 128–133
beans, 21, 26, 27, 33
Be Relaxed programme, 217–219
Bed of Roses, 203
bergamot, 2
berries, 28, 240
betaine, 228
better back programme, 193–197
bicep curls, 119
black pepper aromatherapy oil, 154
blood oranges, 239
blood sugar, 227, 237, 240
body brushing, 66
 Hip and Thigh Detoxifier, 137
body oil recipe, 4
body scan, 142
body scrubs
 Bed of Roses, 203

Citrus Body Glow, 52–53, 75

boiled eggs, 237

breakfast

burning fat, 90

importance of, 20

breastfeeding, micronutrient requirements, 229

breasts, treasuring your, 155

breathing

celebrating spring, 14

rhythmic, 260

brewer's yeast, 232

bridges (yoga), 255

Bright Eyes, 57–58, 75

brow shaping, 269

brown rice, 232

bulimics, micronutrient requirements, 229

buttock squeeze (Pilates), 186

B vitamins, 228, 232

C

calcium supplements, 208

calf stretch, 124

calorie restriction, 236

candles, 222

canned pineapple, 28

capsaicin, 35

carbohydrates

cravings, 91

Glycaemic Index, 87

'little black dress' regime, 286

weight loss, 84

cardiovascular fitness, 107, 108, 109–111

anti-ageing priorities, 263

importance and benefits, 109–110

'little black dress' regime, 287

career changes, 282

Carrying the moon pose, 260

cashew nuts, 232

Cat pose (yoga), 255–256

cellulite solutions

exercise, 134

Hip and Thigh Detoxifer, 137–138

chamomile

aromatherapy oil, 3, 222

teabags, 222

Champneys' light diet plate, 87, 92

Champneys' 'little black dress' regime, 285–287

Champneys' 'sleep deep' plan, 207–209

Champneys' products, 1

Age Excellence Ultimate Hand Treatment, 58

Aqua Therapy Moisture Rich Firming Lotion, 138

Aqua Therapy range, 2, 137, 138, 145

Aqua Therapy Refining Salt Scrub, 137, 145

Chamomile and Rose Moisture Miracle Mask, 203

Citrus Glow Energising Shower Gel, 52

Citrus Glow range, 2, 52

Citrus Sugar Scrub, 52

Cleanse and Purify Refining Mud Mask, 204

Collagen Enriched Anti-Ageing Eye Mask, 271, 273

Collagen Plus Anti-Wrinkle Eye Treatment, 52, 273

Collagen Plus range, 52, 271, 273

Deeply Moisturising Softening Foot Butter, 141

Deep Tissue Toning Massager, 137

Detox Patches, 68

Exotic Bubble Float, 5

Exotic range, 2, 5

Firm and Tone Aromatherapy Oil, 137

Fresh Face Micro-Dermabrasion System, 51, 143, 144, 271

hero products, 5

Intensive Cracked Heel Treatment Balm, 141, 203, 267

Manicure Miracle Softening Scrub, 55

Marine Collagen range, 271

Micro-Dermabrasion Facial Polish, 51, 144

Micro-Dermabrasion System, 51, 143, 144, 271

Moisture Miracle Facial Oil, 204

Moisture Miracle Rescue Balm, 144

Nail and Cuticle Wonder Oil, 59, 143

Natural Micro-Derm Face Polish, 51, 204

Oriental Body Cream, 267

Oriental Body Glow, 267

Oriental range, 3, 267

Oriental Sensual Body Mist, 267

Oriental Shower Cream, 267

Perfect Skin Illuminating Beauty Balm, 144, 204, 273

Perfect Sleep Bath Milk, 78

Perfect Sleep Pillow Mist, 5, 78, 207

Pure Relaxation Massage Oil, 5, 199, 267

Radiance Boosting Foamy Facial Wash, 51, 143, 204
Radiant Skin Double Enzyme Mask, 271
Rose range, 3
Skin Comforting Gentle Cleansing Milk, 143
Skin Conditioning Gentle Toner, 144
Skin Smoothing Rose Body Scrub, 203
Skin Softening Rose Body Wash, 203
Super Calm Lip Balm, 273
Super Cooling Eye Rescue Gel, 204
Super Rich Floral Facial Balm, 204, 222, 272
Ultra Rich Rose Body Butter, 203
Vitamiracle Rejuvenating Hand and Nail Cream, 203
Champneys' restoration day, 217–219
Champneys' spas, ix–x, 48
chest stretch, 123
chicken, 34
chicken soup, 165
Child's pose (yoga), 75, 256
Chinese medicine, 261
Christmas, 285
Citrus Body Glow, 52–53, 75
clear outs, 14
coenzyme Q10, 228
conjugated linoleic acid (CLA) supplementation, 90
contraceptive pill, 229
convalescents, 229, 242
core strength, 262
    'little black dress' regime, 287
Corpse pose (yoga), 256–257
cosmetics makeovers, 79
cranberries, 239
cravings, beating, 237
creating your at-home spa, 1–5
creating your sanctuary, 63
creativity, rediscovering your, 278
cuddling, 222
curl-ups, 118–119
    better back programme, 196
    Pilates, 189

D

dairy products, 21
detoxing
    Champneys' 'little black dress' regime, 285

exercise, 259
    Hip and Thigh Detoxifier, 137–138
    your body, 65–75, 137–138, 259, 285
    your life, 61–62
diagonal stretch, 126
diet, see nutrition and diet
dieters, micronutrient requirements, 229
'disease to please', 214
downward-facing dog (yoga), 256
Drainers, 61, 62
dried fruits, 28

E

Eastern exercises, 259–260
Eastern massage technique, 261
Echinacea, 162
eggs, 237
elongation stretch, 126
emotional eating, 236
endurance, see muscular strength and endurance
Energisers, 61
energy levels (quiz), 7
equipment and products, essential, 3–4
escape
    autumn, 217–219
    Be Active programme, 128–133
    rejuvenation programme, 65–75
    relaxation, 217–219, 285–287
    spring, 65–75
    summer, 129–134
    winter, 285–287
essential equipment and products, 3–4
essential oils, see aromatherapy oils
evenings, reclaiming, 283
exercise
    anti-ageing priorities, 263–264
    autumn, 185–197
    Be Active programme, 128–130
    better back programme, 193–197
    building a routine, 107–133
    cardiovascular, 109–111
    cellulite solutions, 134
    components of fitness, 107
    Eastern practices, 259–260

flexibility, 121–126
holiday workout, 127
intensity, 110
interval training, 110
'little black dress' regime, 286, 287
motivation, 131–133
muscular strength and endurance, 113–119
Pilates, 185–190
precautions, 11, 108, 185, 251, 259
quiz, 7
relaxation, 218
spring, 41–48
starting again after a break, 188
summer, 107–134
TV workout, 262
walking, 41, 44–48
warm-up and stretching routine, 42–43
weight loss, 93
winter, 251–264
yoga, 251–257
exfoliation, 273
   Bed of Roses, 203
   Collagen Enriched Anti-Ageing Facial, 271
   Hip and Thigh Detoxifier, 137
   Spa Heaven Cocoon, 267–268
Express French Manicure, 58–59
Express Pedicure, 143
eyebrow shaping, 269
eye treatment, 57–58, 75

F

face lift, half-hour, 269
facial massage, 57–58, 261, 272–273
facials
   Collagen Enriched Anti-Ageing Facial, 271–273
   Fresh Face Facial, 143–144
   Polish and Purify Facial, 51–52, 74
   Pure Balance Facial, 204
facial steamer, 271
fake tans, 54–55
fasting, 71
fats
   anti-ageing diet, 235
   immune system, 163

weight loss, 89
fears, 280
Festival of Lights, 222
figs, 242
fish, 22, 26
   anti-ageing diet, 235
   immune system, 164
fish oil supplements, 235
flax meal, 235
flaxseed oil, 73
flexibility, 107, 108, 121–126
   anti-ageing priorities, 264
   better back programme, 196–197
   hero stretches, 123–126
   'little black dress' regime, 287
   yoga, 253
flower arranging, 78
folic acid, 228
foot massage, 141, 267
frankincense, 3
free radicals, 26, 227, 235
French manicure, 58–59
Fresh Face Facial, 143–144
front of thigh stretch, 124
frozen fruits and vegetables, 27, 28
fruits, 26, 28
   anti-ageing diet, 231
   canned pineapple, 28
   detox, 73
   dried, 28
   frozen, 28
   immune system, 163
   portions, 20

G

garlic, 166, 172, 233
geranium, 3, 272
ginger, 162, 233
ginseng, 162
gluteal stretch, 197
Glycaemic Index (GI), 87–92
Glycaemic Load (GL), 87
glycosylation, 227
goats' cheese, 174

grains, 21, 26
  detox, 73
grapefruit aromatherapy oil, 2
green tea, 21
  anti-ageing diet, 232
  'little black dress' regime, 286
  weight loss, 90

H

hair conditioning treatments, 202, 203
half-hour face lift, 269
Halloween, 154
hamstring stretch, 196
happiness, reconnecting with, 282
Head in the Clouds, 199–200
head massage, 199–200, 204, 267–268
heel lifts (Pilates), 187
herbal teas, 21, 26, 73
herbs, 233
hero moves, 117–119
hero products, 5
hero stretches, 123–126
herring, 164
hill walking, 48
Hip and Thigh Detoxifier, 137–138
hip flexor stretch, 196–197
hip replacement, 190
hip rolls (Pilates), 189–190
hip stretch, 124
holiday workout, 127
homocysteine, 228
Hot Stone Therapy, 275
hydrogenated fats, 235
hydrotherapy, 145

I

immune system, 160–166, 172, 240
  lymph, 65
  quiz, 161
  supplements, 163
  tonics, 162
inner cleanse, 71
  see also detoxing
inner thighs

Pilates, 190
  stretch, 124
interval training, 110
intimacy, 280
iron-rich foods, 232
irresistibility, 148–149

J

jasmine, 2
juniper, 3
junk sleep, 207

K

kidney, 164
kiwi fruit, 240
kyphosis, 186

L

laughter, 214
lavender, 2
  infusion, 78
lemon water, 74–75
lentils, 21, 26, 243
Leonard, Thomas, 148
Lief, Stanley, 71
light diet plate, 87, 92
Lights, Festival of, 222
'little black dress' regime, 285–287
liver, 164
liver tonic, 66
live yoghurt, 164
lordosis, 186
loved ones, reconnecting with, 280
loving yourself, see spa treatments and pampering
lunges, 117
lycopene, 35
lymphatic system, 65–66
  cellulite, 134

M

mackerel, 164
magnesium supplements, 208
make-up, 79
malnutrition, 160

mandarin aromatherapy oil, 2

manicure, French, 58–59

manual lymphatic drainage (MLD), 66

marching (better back programme), 193

massage

    body, 14, 53, 142, 204, 268

    Bright Eyes, 57–58

    Citrus Body Glow, 53

    Collagen Enriched Anti-Ageing Facial, 272–273

    facial, 57–58, 261, 272–273

    foot, 141, 267

    Head in the Clouds, 199–200

    Hip and Thigh Detoxifier, 137–138

    Hot Stone Therapy, 275

    legs, 137–138

    lymphatic system, 66

    outdoor, 142

    Pure Balance Facial, 204

    Sensual Luxury Foot Massage, 141

    shoulder, neck and head, 199–200, 204, 267–268

    Spa Heaven Cocoon, 267–268

may chang, 2

meat, 26

meditation, 142, 279, 280

menopause, 22

micronutrient depletion, 159–160

Midsummer Day, 78

mineral supplements, *see* multivitamin and

    mineral supplements

monounsaturated fat, 233

Mothers' day, 14

motivation, exercise, 131–133

Mountain pose (yoga), 251–252

mud bath, 79

multivitamin and mineral supplements, 14

    anti-ageing, 228, 235

    Champneys 'sleep deep' plan, 208

    conjugated linoleic acid (CLA), 90

    detox, 72

    immune system, 163

    people who benefit from, 229

muscular strength and endurance, 107, 108, 113–119

    anti-ageing priorities, 263–264

back strengthening exercises, better back programme,

    195–196

hero moves, 117–119

hero stretches, 123–126

importance and benefits, 113, 121

N

nails, French manicure, 58–59

naps, 154, 206, 267

natural live yoghurt, 164

neck stretch, 123

neroli, 2

neutral spine, 114, 185, 195

noodles, 28

Nordic walking, 48

nori seaweed, 232

nut butters, 28, 233

nutrient deficiencies, 159–160

nutrition and diet

    'adding in' healthy foods, 19, 20–22

    anti-ageing, 227–237

    autumn, 159–83

    burning fat, 90

    detox, 71–75

    Glycaemic Index (GI), 87–88, 92

    healthy eating, fundamentals of, 25

    immune system, 160–166

    'little black dress' regime, 285–286, 287

    quizzes, 8, 66–68, 234

    rejuvenation programme, 71–75

    shopping basket, 26–28, 231–233

    spring, 19–39

    summer, 83–105

    weight loss, 84–93

    winter, 227–249

nuts, 22, 26

    anti-ageing diet, 232, 235

    detoxing, 73

O

oats, 164

oblique curls

    better back programme, 196

    Pilates, 189

oils, 26
    aromatherapy, see aromatherapy oils
    detox, 26, 73
    see also olive oil
oily fish, 26
    anti-ageing diet, 235
    immune system, 164
older people, micronutrient requirements, 229
olive oil, 26, 35, 235
    detox, 73
olives, 232
omega 3 fatty acids, 159
omega 9 (monounsaturated fat), 233
onions, 172
ORAC scale, 236, 239
oranges, 239, 240
oregano, 233
organic food, 28
outer hips and buttocks stretch 126

P

palm tree (yoga), 252
pampering, see spa treatments and pampering
parsnips, 241
partially-hydrogenated fats, 235
passion, reconnecting with your, 147
patchouli aromatherapy oil, 3
peace of mind, 142
peanut butter, 233
pedicure, 143
pedometers, 45
pelvic tilts, 186
peppermint, 2
perceived exertion scale, 110
'perfect moments', creating, 151
Pilates, 185–190
    back care, 193
pill, contraceptive, 229
pineapple, canned, 28
pine aromatherapy oil, 222
plank (better back programme), 193–194
playfulness, 78, 280
Polish and Purify Facial, 51–52, 74
pomegranates, 239, 240

portion sizes, 25
post-menopausal women, micronutrient requirements 229
posture, 114
    Alexander Technique, 78
    core strength, 262
    and energy levels, 7
    exercise, 287
    and flexibility, 121
    neutral spine, 114
    walking, 44
power naps, 154, 206
precautions, exercise, 11, 108, 185, 251, 259
pregnancy
    exercise precautions, 108, 185, 251, 259
    lavender aromatherapy oils, 2
    micronutrient requirements, 229
press-ups, 118
probiotics, 72, 164
procrastination, avoiding, 213
products and equipment, essential, 3–4
prone cobra (better back programme), 194
protein
    anti-ageing diet, 231
    craving cycle, beating the, 237
    immune system, 163
    'little black dress' regime, 286
    weight loss, 89
pulses, 21, 26, 27, 33
    detox, 73
Pure Balance Facial, 204

Q

quizzes
    emotional eating, 234
    energy levels, 7
    exercise motivation, 131–132
    immune system, 161
    nutrition, 8
    self-esteem, 148–149
    sleep, 8
    stress levels, 211
    toxic overload, 66–68
    work–life balance, 9

R

rapeseed oil, 26

RDAs (Recommended Daily Allowances), 228

reclaiming evenings, 283

reconnecting
    with happiness, 282
    with loved ones, 280

recuperating people, 229, 242

redbush tea, 21

rejuvenation programme, 65–75

relaxation, 142
    active, 7, 283
    exercise routine, 126
    'little black dress' regime, 285–287
    passive, 283
    restoration day, 217–219
    rhythmic breathing, 260
    stretches, 126
    walking slowly, 62
    yoga benefits, 253

Releasing pose, 259

restoration day, 217–219

rhythmic breathing, 260

rice, 232

rose, 3

rosemary
    anti-ageing diet, 233
    aromatherapy oil, 3, 66

rotation method, time management, 213

S

sacred space, creating your own, 63

salads, 21, 26

salmon, 164

salon tans, 54

salt, 21

sanctuary, creating your own, 63

sandalwood, 3

saturated fats, 235

scrub recipe, 4

sea, harnessing the power of the, 145

sea bass, 35

seasonal foods

spring, 39

summer, 105

autumn, 183

winter, 249

seaweed, 232

seeds, 26
    anti-ageing diet, 235
    detox, 73

selenium, 159, 232

self-discovery, 277–283

self-esteem, 148
    and exercise, 287
    and flexibility, 121
    quiz, 148–149

self tans, 54–55

sensuality, unleashing your, 138

Sensual Luxury Foot Massage, 141

shellfish, 164

shoulder stretch, 123

Siberian ginseng, 162

side twists (Pilates), 190

silicon, 159

single arm row, 118

skin brushing, 66

skin elasticity, 253

sleep, 65
    afternoon naps, 154, 206, 267
    'junk', 207
    'little black dress' regime, 286, 287
    quiz, 8
    'sleep deep' plan, 207–209
    yoga benefits, 253

smokers
    energy levels, 7
    micronutrient requirements, 229

smoothies, 20

soak recipe, 4

soba noodles, 28, 233

social contact, 214, 283

soulmates, 282

soya products, 21
    anti-ageing diet, 231
    'little black dress' regime, 286
    weight loss, 90

Spa Heaven Cocoon, 267–268

spa treatments and pampering

    autumn, 199–209

    Bed of Roses, 203

    Bright Eyes, 57–58

    Citrus Body Glow, 52–53

    Collagen Enriched Anti-Ageing Facial, 271–273

    creation, 1–5

    Express French Manicure, 58–59

    Express Pedicure, 143

    Fresh Face Facial, 143–144

    half-hour face lift, 269

    Head in the Clouds, 199–200

    Hip and Thigh Detoxifier, 137–138

    Hot Stone Therapy, 275

    'little black dress' regime, 287

    Polish and Purify Facial, 51–52

    Pure Balance Facial, 204

    self tans, 54–55

    Sensual Luxury Foot Massage, 141

    'sleep deep' plan, 207–209

    Spa Heaven Cocoon, 267–268

    spring, 51–59

    summer, 137–145

    thalassotherapy, 145

    winter, 267–275

spices, 233

spinal suppleness, 260

spinal twist (yoga), 254–255

spine, neutral, 114, 185, 195

spring, 15–17

    aromatherapy oils, 2

    celebrating, 14

    escape, 65–75

    exercise, 41–48

    nutrition, 19–39

    recipes, 31–38

    spa treatments and pampering, 51–59

    well-being, 61–63

spring cleaning, 62

spring equinox, 15

sprouted seeds, 166

squats, 117, 262

stabilisation exercises, better back programme, 193–195

stability balls, 262

'starring' roles, 277–278

static abs, 186

steamer, facial, 271

strawberries, 103

strength, *see* muscular strength and endurance

strengthening exercises, better back programme, 195–196

stress management, 211–214

    quiz, 211

    yoga, 253

stretches, 42–43, 121–126

    better back programme, 196–197

summer, 79–81

    aromatherapy oils, 2

    celebrating, 78

    escape, 129–134

    exercise, 107–133

    nutrition, 83–105

    recipes, 95–104

    spa treatments and pampering, 137–145

    well-being, 147–151

sunbathers, micronutrient requirements, 229

supplements, *see* multivitamin and mineral supplements

sweet potatoes, 172

swimming exercise (better back programme), 195

T

tans, fake, 54–55

tea, 21, 26

    detox, 73

    ginger, 162

    green, see green tea

    immune system, 162, 165

    weight loss, 90

television workout, 262

thalassotherapy, 145

Thanksgiving, 155

thiamine, 232

thyme, 233

time management, 213–214

tinned beans and pulses, 27

tomatoes, tinned, 27

tonics, immune system, 162

toxic overload quiz, 66–68

trans fats, 235
tricep dips, 119
turmeric, 233
TV workout, 262

U

upper back stretch, 123

V

Valentine's Day, 223, 280
varied diet, 25
vegans, micronutrient requirements, 229
vegetables, 26, 27
    anti-ageing diet, 231
    detox, 73
    frozen, 27
    immune system, 163
    'little black dress' regime, 286
    portions, 20
vegetarians
    lifespan, 236
    micronutrient requirements, 229
vitamin B, 228, 232
vitamin C, 159, 232, 239
vitamin E, 232, 233
vitamin supplements, *see* multivitamin and
    mineral supplements

W

wakame seaweed, 232
walking, 41, 44–48
    beginners' programme, 47
    hill, 48
    Nordic, 48
    slowly, for relaxation, 62
    warm-up and stretching routine, 42–43
wall push-ups, 262
walnuts, 232
warm-up routine, 42–43
    Pilates, 186
Warrior pose (yoga), 252–254
water, 20, 26, 287
    benefits, 11
    detox, 73

lemon, 74–75
'little black dress' regime, 286
watermelon, 103
weight loss, 84–93
    benefits, 86
    myths, 93
    yoga, 253
weight training, 113–114
well-being
    autumn, 211–214
    detoxing your life, 61–62
    lymphatic system, 65–66
    sanctuary, creating your, 63
    self-discovery, 277–283
    spring, 61–63
    stress management, 211–214
    summer, 147–151
    winter, 277–283
wholegrains, 21, 26
    detox, 73
winter, 223–225
    aromatherapy oils, 3
    celebrating, 222
    escape, 285–287
    exercise, 251–264
    nutrition, 227–249
    recipes, 239–248
    spa treatments and pampering, 267–275
    well-being, 277–283
wish lists, 222
work–life balance
    quiz, 9
    see also escape; well-being

Y

ylang-ylang aromatherapy oil, 2
yoga, 75, 251–257
    back care, 193
yoghurt, 164

Recipe index

A

apple, pear and cranberry crumble, 247

asparagus, Parma ham and mozzarella cheese, 98

autumnal apple, pear and blackberry juice, 170

B

baked American cheesecake, 181

baked plum tomato marinated in balsamic vinegar, 98

barbecued Provençal salmon cooked en papillote, 101

beef fillet with Thai green risotto and shiitake mushrooms, 246

beetroot and orange salad, 173

berry booster, 104

blue Bavarian, 102

blueberry porridge, 95

butternut squash soup, 173

butternut squash, feta cheese and parsley patties, 244

C

caramelised Marsala pears, 182

celery, apple and walnut salad with honey and lemon yoghurt, 33

Champneys' fresh yoghurt muesli, 95

Champneys' granola, 171

Champneys' muesli, 31

chargrilled breast of chicken on braised pearl barley with lemon and thyme yoghurt sauce, 34

chicken

    chargrilled breast of chicken on braised pearl barley with lemon and thyme yoghurt sauce, 34

    chicken tagine with sweet potato, carrots and prunes, 244

    grilled chicken with lemon and butter beans, 100

chill-out, 104

Christmas cranberry, blood orange and pomegranate juice, 239

cod fillet on braised Puy lentils, 245

courgette and lemon pilaff, 176

cranberry, blood orange and pomegranate juice, 239

D

detox fibre smoothie, 32

E

eggs

    egg white spinach omelette, 96

    scrambled eggs, smoked salmon and dill, 31

energy smoothie, 169

exotic juice, 103

F

fig, Parma ham and Gorgonzola salad, 242

fillet of beef with Thai green risotto and shiitake mushrooms, 246

finnan haddock, poached, 170

fresh herb soup, 97

G

gateaux of rice pudding with a rhubarb compote, 38

Granny Smith jelly with cinnamon cream, 180

granola, 171

grilled chicken with lemon and butter beans, 100

grilled fillets of red mullet, 99

grilled sea bass with sautéed vegetables with a tomato and onion salsa, 35

H

haddock
    poached, 170
    smoked haddock kedgeree, 240
haricot beans and avocado salad with red pepper salsa, 33

I

individual raspberry and honey crème fraiche pots with
    an oatmeal crumble topping, 102

J

juices
    autumnal apple, pear and blackberry juice, 170
    berry booster, 104
    chill-out, 104
    Christmas cranberry, blood orange and pomegranate
        juice, 239
    exotic, 103
    very special summer smoothie, 104
    watermelon–berry granita, 103

K

kedgeree, smoked haddock, 240

L

lamb
    roast lamb rump steaks, 175
    tapenade-stuffed leg of lamb, 36
lemon and courgette pilaf, 176
lentil dhal, 243

M

mozzarella cheese, asparagus and Parma ham, 98
Mrs Murphy's butternut squash soup, 173
muesli
    Champneys' fresh yoghurt muesli, 95
    Champneys' muesli, 31
    oatmeal muesli bars, 248
mushroom and goat's cheese melt with pesto, 174

O

oatmeal muesli bars, 248
orange and beetroot salad, 173
oven-baked field mushrooms and leeks, 178–9

P

pan-fried fillet of spicy cod on braised Puy lentils, 245
pan-fried scallops with a pea purée, 242
panna cotta, vanilla and orange, 37
Parma ham, asparagus and mozzarella cheese, 98
parsnip, honey and mustard soup, 241
poached finnan haddock, 170
porridge
    traditional Scottish, 239
    warm blueberry porridge, 95

R

raspberry and honey crème fraiche pots with an oatmeal
    crumble topping, 102
red mullet, 99
rice pudding with a rhubarb compote, 38
roast lamb rump steaks, 175

S

saffron, potato and garlic broth, 241
salads
    beetroot and orange, 173
    celery, apple and walnut, 33
    fig, Parma ham and Gorgonzola, 242
    haricot beans and avocado, 33
    scallop, 100
salmon
    barbecued Provençal salmon cooked en papillote, 101
    and herb fishcakes, 177
    spaghetti with smoked salmon, capers and chilli, 36
scallops
    with pea purée, 242
    salad with avocado, mango and chilli, 100
Scottish porridge, 239
scrambled eggs, smoked salmon and dill, 31
sea bass, 35
sliced fig, Parma ham and Gorgonzola salad, 242
smoked haddock kedgeree, 240

smoked salmon, 36
smoothies
    detox fibre smoothie, 32
    energy smoothie, 169
    very special summer smoothie, 104
    vitamin smoothie, 240
soups
    fresh herb soup, 97
    Mrs Murphy's butternut squash, 173
    parsnip, honey and mustard soup, 241
    saffron, potato and garlic broth, 241
    sweet potato, 172
spaghetti with smoked salmon, capers and chilli, 36
spiced apple, pear and cranberry crumble, 247
springs' spring zinger, 32
sweet potato soup, 172

T

tapenade-stuffed leg of lamb, 36
Thai green risotto, 246
traditional Scottish porridge, 239

V

vanilla and orange panna cotta, 37
very special summer smoothie, 104
vitamin smoothie, 240

W

warm blueberry porridge, 95
watermelon–berry granita, 103

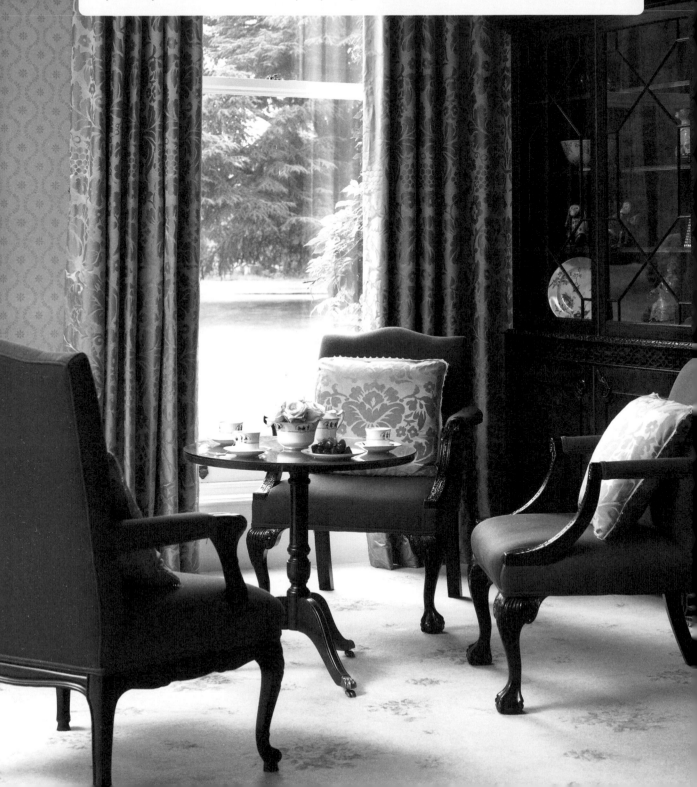

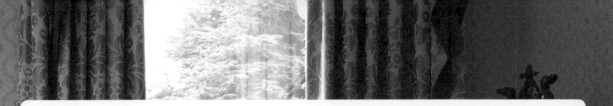
Inspired by some of the tips in this book? Why not visit one of these Champneys resorts to experience first hand the ultimate in pampering and relaxation.

The place to be...

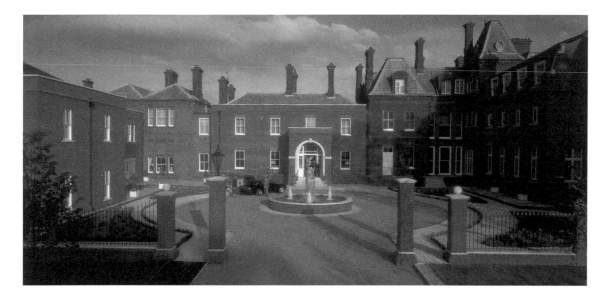

Champneys at Tring

A world-class health resort and spa haven

This elegant English stately home was opened as a health farm in 1925 by the celebrated naturopath Stanley Lief, who pioneered the concept of holistic well-being. Today, Tring remains true to those roots – it is an outstanding health resort in the very heart of Hertfordshire, dedicated to the well-being of your mind, body and soul. A major refurbishment was recently completed, including a state-of-the-art gym and cardio-fitness theatre. Yet the Rothschild Mansion retains its history: take tea, perhaps in the graceful Drawing Room or roam the manicured grounds before an invigorating swim in the new 25-metre pool. After a yoga or Pilates class, flake out with a good book in the warm comfort of your room.

Champneys Tring
Wigginton, Hertfordshire, HP23 6HY • Tel: 01442 291000 • Fax: 01442 291001
For reservations call +44 8703 300 300 or visit www.champneys.com to book your stay today.

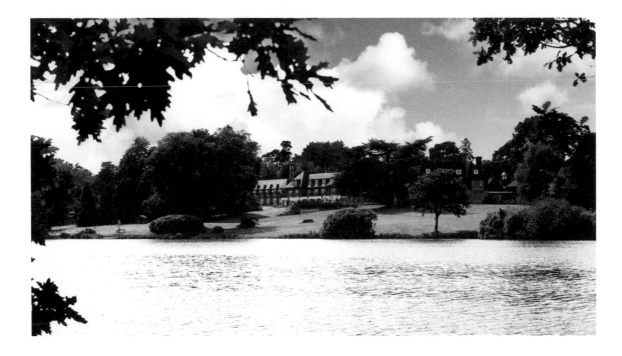

Champneys Forest Mere

Seeing Champneys Forest Mere for the first time is a breathtaking experience.

Beautiful, mysterious woodland leads you to a clearing where the magnificent lake frames the Mansion House. Forest Mere blends enchanting grounds with the latest spa and beauty facilities.

Bathe in the UK's first thalassotherapy pool, take a swim in the 25-metre pool or rejuvenate with mud treatments in the twilight Rasul Chamber. Forest Mere also holds an Alternative Health Clinic where guests can experience a healing circle, and therapies from Reiki to Graphology.

Champneys Forest Mere
Liphook, Hampshire, GU30 7JQ
Tel: 01428 72600 • Fax: 01428 723501

For reservations call +44 8703 300 300 or visit www.champneys.com to book your stay today.

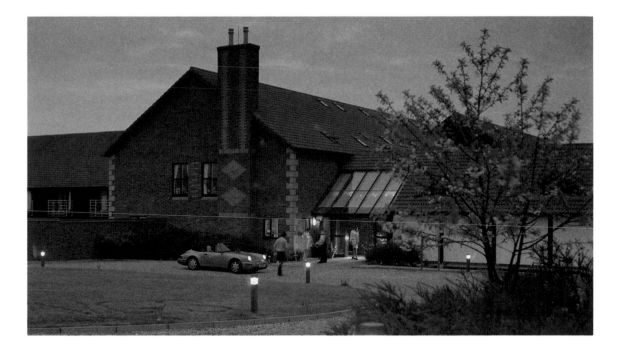

Champneys Springs

Modern luxury with an exceptionally warm friendly service.

Springs was the UK's first purpose built health farm and is now one of the most advanced health spas in the country. As you cross the water walkway with fish swimming below your feet, your worries will just disappear. Surrounded by wide open parklands Springs oozes space and light.

Springs is famous for its friendliness with guests returning time and time again for the welcoming atmosphere. Springs makes a great venue for girly get-togethers, pampering sessions and sporty breaks.

Champneys Springs
Ashby de la Zouch, Leicestershire, LE65 1TG
Tel: 01530 273873 • Fax: 01530 270987

For reservations call +44 8703 300 300 or visit www.champneys.com to book your stay today.

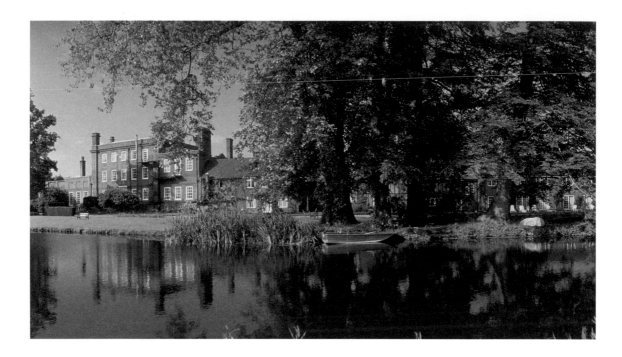

Champneys Henlow

An impressive Georgian mansion nestling in 100 acres of peaceful countryside.

Henlow Grange has over 40 years of history as a health resort and has been a centre of peace for centuries. Henlow Grange has recently completed a major renovation and the new facilities include a Laconium, a herbal steam chamber and two fitness studios. A state of the art Rasul mud chamber and thalassotherapy pool are also available. All bedrooms have been refurbished and even the modern standard rooms are equipped with a flat screen TV and DVD player.

Henlow Grange is decorated in the finest Georgian style, with opulent upholstered furniture, hand painted walls and Venetian style mirrors. Henlow Grange's charm lies in its reverence to the past whilst providing the latest spa facilities. Soak up the atmosphere of another time and way of life and bathe in the beauty that is Henlow Grange.

Champneys Henlow
Henlow, Bedfordshire, SG16 6BD
Tel: 01462 811111 • Fax: 01462 815310

For reservations call +44 8703 300 300 or visit www.champneys.com to book your stay today.

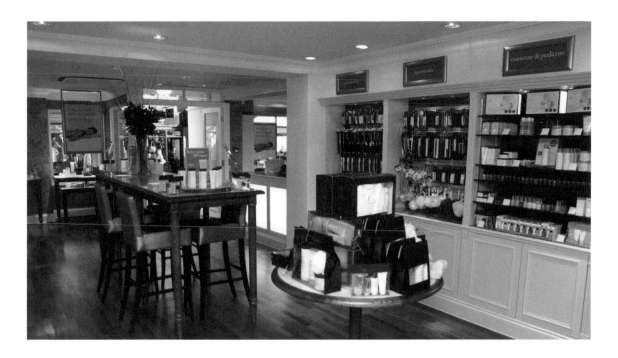

Champneys town and city spas

Whether you have a moment in your lunch hour to maintain your manicure, an hour to de-stress, or maybe an afternoon to completely unwind and relax, Champneys now provide the perfect environment where you can immerse yourself in relaxing surroundings and indulge in a little spa therapy at a location near you. From restored listed buildings in Guildford and St Albans, to the new shopping development in Enfield, Champneys' latest Town and city spas are found in the heart of some of the best shopping locations.

Champneys Chichester
60 East Street, Chichester,
West Sussex. PO19 1HL
Tel: 01243 819010
chichester@champneys.com

Champneys Guildford
194 High Street, Guildford.
Surrey, GU1 3H
Tel: 01483 455850
guildford@champneys.com

Champneys Enfield
Unit 2, Hatton Walk,
Palace Exchange, Enfield EN2 6BP
Tel: 0208 363 7994
enfield@champneys.com

Champneys St Albans
23 Market Place, St Albans
Hertfordshire, AL3 5DP
Tel: 01727 864893
stalbans@champneys.com

Champneys Tunbridge Wells
7 High Street, Tunbridge Wells
Kent, TN1 1UL
Tel: 01892 530111
tunbridgewells@champneys.com

Champneys Brighton
24 East Street, Brighton
East Sussex, BN1 1HL
Tel: 01273 777155
brighton@champneys.com

Champneys Bath
20 New Bond Street, Bath
Somerset, BA1 1BD
Tel: 01225 420 500
bath@champneys.com